Embrace Tiger, Return to Mountain

—the essence of T'ai Chi

Al Chung-liang Huang

BANTAM BOOKS · TORONTO · LONDON · NEW YORK

This low-priced Bantam Book
has been completely reset in a type face
designed for easy reading, and was printed
from new plates. It contains the complete
text of the original hard-cover edition.
NOT ONE WORD HAS BEEN OMITTED.

❧

RLI: $\dfrac{\text{VLM 5 (VLR 4-7)}}{\text{IL 8+}}$

EMBRACE TIGER, RETURN TO MOUNTAIN
*A Bantam Book / published by arrangement with
Real People Press*

PRINTING HISTORY
Real People edition published January 1974
2nd printing . . . April 1974
Bantam edition / May 1978

ISBN 0-553-02571-6

Published simultaneously in the United States and Canada

Bantam Books are published by Bantam Books, Inc. Its trade-
mark, consisting of the words "Bantam Books" and the por-
trayal of a bantam, is registered in the United States Patent
Office and in other countries. Marca Registrada. Bantam
Books, Inc., 666 Fifth Avenue, New York, New York 10019.

PRINTED IN THE UNITED STATES OF AMERICA

水 鏡
花 月

Water — mirror
moon — flower

To
my parents and my daughter
and
most of all
To
my wife
Suzanne

Contents

A Fresh Note to Introduce This New Edition

Tao is still alive, living in all of us. It is alive in me, in all of my personal daily involvements. Essentially, the T'ai Chi I practiced and talked about is still ever-constant, and ever-changing. From time to time, an ex-pupil would appear in my workshop and exclaim: "But, you have changed this . . ." My answer has been, "No, I have not. I move on and beyond . . . but you got stuck back then and there." My variations of teaching continue to develop and transform, but the essence is the same. Tao is still mysterious and ineffable. It continues to reveal to us in many ways: in the hidden fragrance of a lone orchid in deep mountain, in windflow and watercourse ways, and in the simplest effortlessness of fish in water and bird in flight. Above all, it is in all of us when we become an active participant in living, instead of being merely an observer of life. My second daughter Tysan at two years is the new t'ai chi master in the Huang family. She still has the quintessence! And Lark, the little buddha sitting transfixed at dawn in Harry Steven's cave I wrote about in the Afterword, is ready to enter first grade. These days some of my t'ai chi disciples are climbing trees, rolling down the hills, and flying kites with them. Juggling while gliding on Lark's skateboard is still a challenge to me. But Tysan always applauds encouragingly each time I fall . . .

Happy reading and moving joyously too,

AL CHUNG-LIANG HUANG

Summer's end and a new
Autumn in the Middle-west
1976

Foreword

My association with the author of this book is not simply that I have read his work and like it. We have known each other for quite a number of years. We have jointly conducted seminars at Esalen Institute and similar places, where I have spoken of Taoist philosophy and he has demonstrated its place in terms of t'ai chi movement. We have spent much time together exploring this venerable philosophy, both intellectually and practically, and have come to a consensus of understanding and feeling about it such that I can say of the relationship betwen us that East and West have undoubtedly met—and, for me, this is no small matter.

To begin with, Huang teaches in a way that is unusual for an Asian master and, when I think back over my own schooling, for Western masters as well. He begins from the center and not from the fringe. He imparts an understanding of the basic principles of the art before going on to the meticulous details, and he refuses to break down the t'ai chi movements into a one-two-three drill so as to make the student into a robot. The traditional way (whether in t'ai chi, zen, or yoga) is to teach by rote, and to give the impression that long periods of boredom are the most essential part of training. In that way a student may go on for years and years without ever getting the feel of what he is doing. This is true of theology, law, medicine, and mathematics as it is of t'ai chi, so that we have many "masters" of these disciplines who are plainly incompetent, no more than well-contrived imitations of the real thing. The strengths and weaknesses of human nature are the same in Asia as in the West: there are plenty of Buddhist, Hindu, and Taoist equivalents of pompous bishops, knife-happy surgeons, and pedantic scholars who cannot see the forest for the trees.

T'ai chi exemplifies the most subtle principle of Taoism, known as wu-wei. Literally, this may be translated as "not doing," but its proper meaning is to act without forcing—to move in accordance with the flow of nature's course which is signified by the word Tao, and is best understood from watching the dynamics of water. Wu-wei is exemplified in the art of sailing, in which one uses intelligence, as distinct from rowing, in which force of muscle is dominant. In such arts as sailing, gliding, surfing, and skiing there must be no turns through sharp angles, for in such sharp turns human muscle would have to defy the environment of water, wind, or gravity instead of using it.

The spirit of wu-wei is to make turns with curves instead of crick-crack angles, and for this reason the whole biological world is curvaceous—water being its main component. As Lao-tzu said, although water is soft and weak it invariably overcomes the rigid and hard. To work with Huang is to learn to move with wind and water—not only in the t'ai chi exercises, but also in the course of everyday life. In going by "the watercourse way" he is as fresh as a mountain stream, with all its bubbles and babbles, and, way down below, as deep and powerful as the Yang-tze Chiang.

Too many masters of the arts of life are disciplinary martinets, perhaps because too many of their students, while thinking that they ought to learn, do not really want to. All compulsory education is forced growth, and produces tasteless fruit. But with his skill in t'ai chi, as well as in dancing and flute-playing, Huang Chung-liang woos and beguiles his students instead of forcing them. This is the mark of a truly superior and gifted teacher who works upon others as the sun and rain upon plants.

ALAN WATTS

Druid Heights,
Rancho Saucelito, California
1973.

Introduction

There are no beginnings and no endings. The universe is process and the process is in me. When I fight this process or ignore it, I am in trouble. When I move with it, something happens—like this book. My part in it is small. That doesn't make it unimportant. Arbitrarily, I choose a beginning for the process of this book.

At Esalen, two and a half years ago, a friend said, "Have you seen Al Huang? He's great!" I hadn't. "He is visiting here and he does t'ai chi on the deck an hour before lunch." I had sometimes enjoyed watching t'ai chi—as with Master Choy in Berkeley—and sometimes not—as with people whose joints seemed to go "click!" as they switched from one position to another like mechanical dolls. I had no interest in learning t'ai chi. The next morning I was out on the deck. Al told us to walk "as if you don't know what's there—maybe it's grass, maybe it's water." When I did this, tentativeness came into my body and released my mind from its clutching certainty. We held imaginary soap bubbles in our hands and walked with them. Hold them too tight, they break. Hold them too loose, they slip away.

I told Steve. Next day, he was there, too. All three of us were immediately close in the bubble-touching way, with exceptional delight, that happens seldom. We spoke with Al about the possibility of doing a book about his work, but initially Al was reluctant, saying "What I do is the doing," and doubting that anything in print could convey much of the spirit of his work. As an experiment, we taped a week-long workshop at Esalen in July, 1971, and later transcribed it. Al liked the transcript, so we used the material from this workshop as a framework for this book, editing, expanding sections, and adding material from transcripts of other workshops. The photographs were taken by Si Chi Ko, a photographer friend of Al's, during a workshop at the Roscoe Center in New York in the spring of 1973. So the book has slowly grown over the past two and a half years in a very t'ai chi way. Even now, as the book is in galley proofs, it is still growing. Al writes:

"I have thought of several things that we have talked about but not included in the book. I have been noting them down, using them during workshops last month. But it will always be ongoing, changing, with new discoveries day-to-day.

"*Energy* is a confusing term. I try to make it clear that it is not nervous tension and not phony mental wishing. It is subtle and powerful, and circulates continuously in one's mental/physical self. Acupuncture's meridians show the paths of this ch'i-energy. In practicing t'ai chi ch'uan, as in pushing forward in the fire-element step, what one senses is the circular path of the ch'i from tant'ien out through the palms of the hands, outward and curving around to return to center. Beginners can only imagine it, and feel it fragmentedly. After long years of practice, it becomes very obvious. Energy is open, free-moving, unburdened, basically undefinable. It is life-force unforced, which then becomes forceful and powerful.

"*Flow* is so overused as a word. It sometimes suggests loosely letting go, sloppy, mushy, self-indulgent 'freedom' which is really not true spontaneity. Flow is like blood circulation, or breathing easily without self-consciousness. The ch'i flows in the body meridians when a body is perfectly healthy and natural. A person can't force flow. Flow flows until we block it.

"After the first day of t'ai chi, one man went home bumping into things, feeling particularly clumsy. His first thought was negative: 'How come t'ai chi is not making me graceful and flowing better?' Then he realized that all his life he had been living and moving only partially and with constriction. Now, in spite of himself, he was moving bigger. His ch'i took over and he couldn't keep up with it, so he found his usual space too cramped, bumped into things, and felt slightly disoriented.

"Last month I worked with a one-armed woman, a man with his right gluteus minumus muscle removed, and another man with a braced leg. The discovery for all of us was that the ch'i moves beyond the physical body. If we learn to relate to our tant'ien, and move beyond our physical limitations, without relying on muscles, we discover the simplest way to stay centered. By the end of the week, the woman was spinning and feeling balanced, and the men walked and danced without their crutches."

In order to make a book we have to stop this changing growth process somewhere and set down what we have in unchanging print. Steve writes:

"T'ai chi is a subtle and powerful awareness discipline, a tool to become more in touch with yourself. It is a way of allowing yourself to function naturally and smoothly, uncluttered with expectations, shoulds, hopes, fears, and other fantasies that interfere with our natural flow. Unlike so many paths to awareness, t'ai chi is beautiful to experience as you do it, and also beautiful to watch from the outside.

"Besides the utility and beauty of t'ai chi in itself, it has been valuable to me as an embodiment and expression of the psychological processes that I see in gestalt therapy work. If I continually reach out to others for love, I am tipping forward, off-center and unstable, leaning on whoever I contact, and likely to fall flat and hard if the other leaves. If I continually withdraw in fear, I am tipping backward, tense and rigid, and the slightest surprise will push me over. If I feel uncertain in myself and unstable in my base, then all my contacts with others will be wobbly and lack conviction. In contrast, if I can become centered and balanced in my own experience, then I can carry this moving center with me. If I am balanced *now*, then

I can move in any direction I wish with no danger of falling, and my contact with you is solid and real, coming to you from the root of my living.

"I could write much more. But this is Al's book. He is a teacher who is living what he is doing, unpretentiously and with great clarity, beauty, and aliveness."

Steve relates t'ai chi to human relations. Alan Watts writes of surfing and skiing. How about our daily lives? In Moab, Utah, there is a t'ai chi short order cook who has never heard of t'ai chi. It's beautiful to watch him make hamburgers. In Albuquerque, I knew a t'ai chi mailman. My father was a North of England peasant who went to London and learned a trade. He taught me to do everything without force. "Easy does it," weren't just words to him. "If you have to force it, then something's wrong. Find out what it is." When I was sixteen, he taught me to drive a car, first briefly telling me the simple mechanics. After that he sat beside me while I drove, saying "*Listen* to the gears. Listen to the sound of tires on the road. Listen to the engine, and smell it, too. Don't expect the road around the bend to be the way you think it is. Don't expect the driver of the car ahead to make sense—maybe he's a lunatic." Be aware, alert and sensing, living and moving in harmony, with no grinding and no crash.

A young Indian working for the Forest Service, cutting trails in mountainous country, said he didn't understand the way the other young men worked. "They attack the brush with such force—and then they sit down and puff and pant. Then they fight it again—and sit down and rest again." He demonstrated their actions with his body, and then his own way. His own way was easy t'ai chi flowing movements, swinging and returning without a break—strength without force. "I don't have to rest," he said, "I can do that all day."

When we were doing t'ai chi with Al's class in Provo, Utah, a man watched us for ten or fifteen minutes. He had never seen ta'i chi before and asked what it was. "That would be good for athletes," he said, "and for my mother's arthritis."

This sounds like I'm calling t'ai chi a panacea—and it is. T'ai chi is zen, is dhyana, is meditation, is yoga, is gestalt—and you have to put them all in a circle and start anywhere to know that. *Panacea* means simply "to cure all." No promise of *instant* cure, or that someone can do it to or for you, or that some pill will do it. Unlearning what has been going on for centuries is not easy, and ego/intellect/I rebels at giving up control and taking second place—the function it was designed for. It's a radical change, and ego screams that it's all nonsense, and babbles of the terrible things that will happen to me if I do it. Al Huang's way of teaching lets me experience something and know that I feel good with it. Ego says "Yes, but . . . ." I learn a little, and forget a lot. In our society, sometimes I feel as if I'm trying to learn to ride a bicycle and people and events and requirements keep throwing me. This happens to Al Huang too. In a letter written in April, he said:

"Days like that: When I must be on time to teach the t'ai chi class, and Lark is fussy, making unreasonable demands to slow down the process, and as a result I run right past a stop sign and get a ticket.

"Moments like this one: When I just finished suggesting to a student not to rush life, to enjoy the process and look at the trees and clouds between running from place to place, I turned around and tripped down the staircase. Irony or paradox? Innocence or fake belief? Charlatan in all of us? Part of it, often all of it, is true. And because of it, we can laugh and ring clear and release ourselves to be more free.

"I suppose the whole idea of being called a t'ai chi Master, and a prospective author on the subject of life's dimensions, puzzles me. I am conscious of the burden. And subconsciously delaying the process of buckling down to complete the manuscript."

Last week, in the isolated desert valley where I live, it had been 100 degrees or more for a couple of weeks. Then it rained. I steamed. I wished for the shower that I didn't want to take because we're having water supply problems. I would be stoic. Like concrete. Then I woke up, took off my clothes, and went for a walk in the rain.

BARRY STEVENS,
JOHN STEVENS

Shura, Utah
1973.

Embrace Tiger,
Return to Mountain

I

It happens: We sit here in a circle in silence. Most of the time we find it very difficult to sit and not break the silence . . . and just allow something to happen.

I'm not here to teach you anything. I'm here to share with you how I learn about t'ai chi. So hopefully by the end of the week you will begin to learn about t'ai chi through *you*. T'ai chi is just a Chinese word for something that appears in many forms of discipline. Yoga, in essence, is t'ai chi. Zen is t'ai chi. T'ai chi is what is. No more, no less.

Some of you have learned the *form* of t'ai chi ch'uan. We will practice some of the forms and we will work on them, but my main purpose is to help you to recreate what happened many hundreds of years ago when the taoists first created t'ai chi ch'uan. What happened then? What was that creative process that made it such a spontaneous form that even now we look at this phrase of movement and say, "Ah, that's beautiful, that's so simple, and I can identify with it." And then when you begin to learn, it's so hard, because you're fighting between the structure and what seems to be so unattainable.

There is a lot of confusion about what t'ai chi is, and what t'ai chi *ch'uan* is. Mostly everybody is concerned with what form is being done. "Oh, I study from so and so, and he studies from Master Tsung— or Master Choy—and this is the Ma style and this is

1

the Wu style and this is the Yan style. What do you practice?" I say "I practice the Huang style." My style comes out of all these other styles, and I have to develop to the point that it becomes me.

I discovered t'ai chi first as a child, completely unprejudiced. Out in the field every morning, the t'ai chi master would practice, and we would follow and have fun with ourselves. We had years and years of working this way with the master, and before we knew it we were doing it, and it had become ours. I lost it when I came to this country, and then I had to work backward and recapture it after I became a concert dancer. I found that the only way I can really keep my movement and my dancing fresh is to work within myself in the t'ai chi way—which is a constant re-creation, a regeneration of energy and a re-birth each time I do it. This is why t'ai chi is so vital for movement and dance, where you really work with your body.

In this culture, we rely so much on the mind that we become separated from other aspects of our living. An exercise, a discipline like t'ai chi immediately points out where you lack, where you go astray. Why do you find something that is so easy to understand intellectually, so difficult to do? This division between thinking and doing is so clear; it takes so long to really find that yin/yang balance.

The yin/yang symbol is the interlocking, melting together of the flow of movement within a circle. The similar—and at the same time obviously contrasting— energies are moving *together*. Within the black area there is a white dot and within the white fish shape, there is a black dot. The whole idea of a circle divided in this way is to show that within a unity there is duality and polarity and contrast. The only way to find real balance without losing the centering feeling of the circle is to think of the contrasting energies moving together and in union, in harmony, interlocking. In a sense this is really like a white fish and a black fish mating. It's a union and flowing interaction.

It's a kind of consummation between two forces, male and female, mind and body, good and bad. It's a very important way of living. People identify with this kind of concept in the Orient much more than in our Western culture, where the tendency is to identify with one force and to reject the contrasting element. If you identify with only one side of the duality, then you become unbalanced. T'ai chi can help you to realize how you are unbalanced and help you to become centered again as you re-establish a flow between the two sides. So don't get stuck in a corner, because a circle has no corners. If you think in this way, you open up more, and you don't feel like you have to catch up with anything.

Someone said that the difference between an Oriental man and a Western man is this: The Oriental man is very empty and light up here in the head and very heavy down here in the belly and he feels very secure. The Western man is light in the belly and very heavy up here in the head, so he topples over. In our Western society so much is in the head, so much is in talking and thinking about things, that we can analyze everything to pieces and it's still distant from us, still not really understood. We have so many mechanical gadgets to do our work for us that our bodies are underemphasized. In order to regain balance we have to emphasize the body and we must work with the mind-body together.

Some people realize that their bodies need more work, so they run, jog, ride bicycles, swim, and then say "O.K. I have done my share of exercise." But this is still a separation of "body time" and "mind time," like the separation of work and play that most people experience. You work very hard so that you can take a vacation and come to a beautiful place to enjoy yourself. This brings a separation in your life. Working shouldn't be such a chore. Playing shouldn't be such a straining for fun, fun, fun. Work and play can combine. Nonverbal activities are a very important way to regain balance and find unity in your life.

When you stop talking you have a chance to open up and become receptive to what is happening in your body and to what is going on around you.

T'ai chi is one of the many ways to help you to discipline your body and find a way to release that tension within you. T'ai chi can be a way of letting your body really teach you and be with you and help you to get through the conflicts you encounter every day.

As a movement teacher, as a t'ai chi teacher, I find the most difficult thing is an *un*learning process that we have to go through. So the first couple of days we will be unlearning.

There is a lovely story about a professor who comes to a zen master. He says, "Hello, I'm doctor so and so, I'm such and such. I would like to learn from you about Zen Buddhism." The master says, "Would you like to sit down?" "Yes." "Would you like some tea?" "Yes." He pours some tea, and he continues pouring even after the cup is full, and finally the professor says, "The tea is spilling all over, it is spilling all over!" And the master says, "Exactly. You come with a full cup. Your cup is already spilling over, so how can I give you anything? You are already overflowing with all that knowledge. Unless you come with emptiness and openness, I can give you nothing." We need that kind of innocence, that kind of ignorance, in learning and dealing with things every day.

So we will have to practice emptying our cups to allow us to receive. We were doing some of this as we were sitting here in silence. In a way we were emptying our thoughts and anticipations. Each of you comes with a different kind of expectation. Some of you know my work; some of you think it's going to be good for you. For others, this is just a try. You all have different kinds of anticipations of what you want, and it will take a few sessions for us to really settle down and just be with ourselves *now* in working.

Sitting in a circle is such a simple way of saying that I'm you and you and you and you, and we are the circle, we are here. Right there is the center. While I'm talking, I'm using verbal thoughts to communicate with you but what I'm really doing is sensing you. This also gives me time to empty my own cup of what I want to say—my anxiety to get across to you what t'ai chi is. It's so easy for me to say and so hard for me to get *to* you. And sooner or later we reach a dead end when we talk.

So what we have to do is go back and forth between talk and experience. We will talk for a while, and then experiment with movement. I like to start my own meditation practice as early as possible, and t'ai chi works very well in the early morning. But because of the hours we keep here at Big Sur, and the reluctance to go to bed, if we begin to dance and enjoy the baths and the moon, we usually don't get to bed as early as we should. Because of the mountain, the sun comes up very late, about seven o'clock now. I will begin practicing by the pool around seven-thirty, and I would like all of you to come and join me. Tonight, before we finish, I will provide you with some structure and motifs for you to do. But in the morning, I do not speak: I do not talk to you; you do not talk to me. And you should not watch me and say, "Let's do what he does." You each do your own t'ai chi.

Those of you who have studied t'ai chi from another master, don't say, "Let's compare this: this is not quite the same," or "He is doing that first, I'm doing that last." T'ai chi is an individual discipline; it's not the kind of unison movement you find in a set choreography.

One of the best images for t'ai chi is nature, and the movement of nature. The different branches on the same tree do not move the same but they are moving in unity. When you look at nature, everything has its own motion: the tree and the rock and the water running—they somehow tie together without making a point to fit. When you watch the waves coming over the rocks, you see that the wave has wave-nature, rock has rock-nature. They do not violate each other's nature. That's a tao concept, a zen concept that exactly fits into t'ai chi practice.

In the evenings, we will have an open movement session with live music. We will do some folk dancing. I have also brought some tapes which are a result of my t'ai chi sessions with some musicians that I've worked with. So we can work through different ways to get to the same process.

Now there is change. Our circle just expanded because of the new people joining in. Understanding t'ai chi makes you feel like an amoeba. That's something we have to do: We have to return to being an amoeba, so we can recapture our resilience. There are always these two elements: You wish you could dance like somebody else, and you wish you could still move like a child. You look at children or you look at somebody who happens to be a very fine mover or dancer and you say, "That's very graceful, that's very nice." And I would say you can do the same thing. You may not be able to kick your leg as high as someone else, but that's not the point. That's only a particular extension, a particular achievement.

The basic process in movement is a sense of *awareness*, and a sense of *being*. When you feel like you're together, you're dancing. When you are not dancing is when you feel like you are "all over the place." Your mind is thinking here, your muscle tensed up there; you do not know where you are any more, and suddenly you trip over something and hurt yourself. Being together means centering, means t'ai chi.

This is all intellectual so far—we all understand this. Those of you who come here, you already have some positive sense of what you want—to be *more* with yourself. You want to *extend* more, you want to *come back* more, you want to just *feel* more—with your whole total being: body and mind moving together. And I would say do more with the body. Most of us are heavy enough up here in the head, so let's get down here, in the body.

All right. Let's stand up where we are now. Tonight I just want to point out some simple, obvious things that we can do. When you are standing up, you are nothing but muscles holding your bones. What is important is *how* you are holding up this structure. My daughter is one year old; she's just walking. It's a marvel to watch her having so much fun squatting down and standing up—a real discovery with her body. We usually take most of this for granted, and at other times we try too hard to hold ourselves up.

One way of loosening up is by shaking yourself all over. In this kind of shaking you sometimes do too much, and become more tense. I want you to extend this shaking movement and at the same time just let everything go. If you still feel tension, try to simply become more aware of your tension, and go with it. Sometimes this takes a little longer, but it really is a better way. If you shake yourself, you are still *doing* something with your body instead of *allowing* it to happen. When you shake yourself you sometimes become more tense. Letting go by just becoming aware of tension is an example of wu wei—doing by not doing, non-assertion, non-interference. So in the beginning it is useful to simply accept what your body is doing. When you really accept your tension, letting go will happen without effort and you will become less tense. All your life you've been told, "Stand up on your own two feet. Take care of yourself. Be responsible. Hold the world on your shoulders." You try so hard to stand up straight, to be strong and not to crumble, not to give in, not to be a failure, not to do the wrong thing.

Right now, allow your body to let go while remaining in a standing position. Become really aware of what gravity is doing to you, and go along with that. It's not a matter of being crushed down and crumbling. Just let gravity pull you down and help you let go. Give in to this force. You don't have to be either weak or strong.

If I go around and push down on your shoulders, you should bounce with me like a ping-pong ball. The basic thing is to realize how tight we are, just standing up. No matter how free we *think* we want to be, it is still often just in our minds. The mental freedom and the physical freedom are soon separated. This is why we need the body awareness and discipline. The whole idea of this kind of technique is first an acceptance, and then a willingness to give in, and then a discipline to help you find a constant understanding of this living balance in your body.

Usually in my beginning sessions when I push down on your shoulders, almost everybody makes me work very hard, until you realize how unnecessary it is to fight back. Your body has the curves and bends to give in, to be resilient in your ankles, knees, hips and shoulders. When we realize that all this holding up is unnecessary, and all this tightening and rigidity is not needed, then we can bounce again.

The second time I come around to push you down, it is usually a little easier for you to give. Now you can sense how much energy I push with; you can go with me, and somehow we are rhythmically in tune. It's an easy feeling. Now your body doesn't need to hold up so straight. The body is made with these marvelous joints which bounce and recoil. One of the best images of zen and tao is to be like bamboo, or a bow. You can feel the weight here on your shoulders. But instead of resisting, you bend like a bow and then spring back when the weight releases. Instead of resisting the energy, you store it up and use it as you recoil.

Now stretch your arms up over your head. Get hold of your hands and stretch to your full length. Keep stretching and think of this energy going up. Then let your hands come apart; let your arms just flow out and down to your sides. You can sense how this upward energy moves out and down in a circle. The length of your arm becomes the curve of a ball and your energy shoots out and down. Now experience the relief of that feeling in your neck and chest when you let your arm go, and enjoy the descent.

When energy stores inside of us without natural release, we build up tension. Since energy is a continuous source of being alive every day, we must learn to be with it, to release it when necessary and to regenerate it. This time when your hands release, try to let the body also settle down; let your knees go a little bit, and sink.

Some of you begin to forget to breathe. When you release your arms, release that air too and let it come out. You can begin to discover the natural coordination of your inhalation/exhalation that corresponds with this simple gesture of stretching, and then letting go and descending.

As you do it several times, you also notice that the hands have to break when they do. You do not plan to break. When the hands have to break, they break. Those of you who have read Herrigel's *Zen in the Art of Archery* know the imagery when he writes that "the arrow lets go." When it's ready to shoot, it will go and the energy will aim for the bulls-eye. The bulls-eye is not a fixed place. It only appears as the energy gathers, ready to be sent forth. What you can feel is the release in your chest, and the sensation of the air flowing out. Unless the whole body allows this giving in to it, you can't be sure of the release of the chest and the whole feeling of letting the air just flow out. Inhale as you reach up and clasp your hands together and stretch, and then let the air flow out as your hands break apart and flow down. Let your whole body sink a little as your arms come down.

Now let the downward movement flow continuously into an upward movement, so that you don't lose the energy. As your hands come down, let them come in and then scoop up in front of you as you reach up again.

Just try this for fun. I'm going to give you three counts up, three counts down. When you get into a regular rhythm like this, it makes you feel somewhat mechanical. Because of our individual differences in height, because of our own differing sense of expansion and contraction, we are varying in spite of our efforts to stay with the count. Those of you who are familiar with the Eastern or Hindu music know that the whole rhythmical structure is quite different from most conventional Western music which depends on the bar-line structure. Many contemporary musicians try to get out of this rigid confinement by doing away with bar-lines and by mixing meters. This music gets back to a more natural flow that corresponds with the emotional and bodily changes.

This is why in t'ai chi practice we do not count: We work on a continuous flow. This is another aspect of t'ai chi, which ties in exactly with the *I Ching*, the *Book of Changes*. Change is yin and constant is yang, or vice versa. So the constant thing is that we all can fit into the changing rise and fall. The change is constant; the constant is change. In movement, we learn to really understand this intellectual concept. Part of our everyday conflict is how to cope with the changes and how to be happy with the constant. We are usually bored with the constant, and we get frantic with the change. We have all kinds of gimmicks: "Meditate!" "Pull yourself together!" "Relax!" "Do therapy!" But these all boil down to one thing: Accept *both* the constant and the change. Learn how to be resilient and responsive to your surroundings, to time, and to yourself.

In t'ai chi practice, you move very slowly. By moving very slowly you have time to be aware of all the subtle details of your movement and your relationship to your surroundings. It's so slow that you really have no way of saying this is slower than that or faster than that. You reach a level of speed that is like slow motion, in which everything is just happening. You slow it to the point that you are fully involved in the process of each moment as it happens. You transcend the form and any concern you might have to achieve some particular motif.

It's like when we were sitting here very silently and you were waiting for me to start. You were wondering, "When is he going to begin?" Everybody is getting tense. You keep wondering and waiting, and after a while you realize there's no use wondering. "He'll start whenever he wants to start, and I'll just relax." Some of you begin to relax. Suddenly time stands still for a second. There's a moment when you are willing to say, "Let it happen, whatever happens, whenever it's happening." "It's not my worry, I don't have to push it or rush it." You allow that moment to happen.

The same is true for me. If I worry, if I am self-conscious, I must first allow that tension to go, and then I will begin. I may have a whole bunch of things stuffed in my mind that "I have to get across to you tonight," but if I don't just drop it and let it all go, it will never come out right. I will just be reciting what I have written down. Or I will just tell you all about t'ai chi history and concepts. Most of you have read about this already, and intellectually you understand —there's no need for me to repeat it. What happens tonight must grow out of what we feel now.

I came here a little earlier on Friday, to sit in on the last two sessions of an aikido workshop. They were working on sensing and the feeling of balance. Aikido is an outgrowth of t'ai chi, created by Morihei Uyeshiba less than a hundred years ago in Japan. Aiki means the unity, the gathering of the ki. The Japanese ki is the same as the ch'i, the breath essence of t'ai chi. The do in the word aikido is the same as tao, the path or the way. Aikido means the way of unifying your ch'i.

There are many other outgrowths of t'ai chi. Judo means "the gentle way." Karate means "the empty hand." Kendo and kenpo are Japanese sword practices which also developed out of the same basic principles. All of these are extensions and developments of the t'ai chi foundation, and all are based on the sense of meditation and movement, flow and awareness.

All these Japanese forms of movement and center-ing are very highly developed forms of t'ai chi. The Japanese forms developed out of Zen Buddhism, which came from the Chinese Ch'an Buddhism. Ch'an Buddhism developed out of the union between Hindu mysticism and Chinese Taoism. Two major forms are exclusively Chinese. One is the t'ai chi ch'uan; the other is kung-fu, which literally means "the skillful man—the man's skill, his energy skill." It's commonly used to mean various series of exercises that show how strong you can be, that you know how to fight. Kung-fu is a very masculine, aggressive, yang way of extending your t'ai chi energy. Judo and aikido use the contrasting receptive yin approach, self-protection rather than aggression. T'ai chi is both yin and yang; it is the center pole, right in the middle. With t'ai chi as a basis you can move easily into any of these different extensions.

Important to all of these is the sense of balance, and the feeling of knowing where you are. Most of you have some sense of where your center is, physically. When you sit, you try to find a comfortable position. In a way you are trying to find your center so you can be more settled and comfortable. In Zen Buddhist zazen when you sit in lotus position, you find your center. In hatha yoga postures you also put your body into a closer position so you can really sense where you are. All these ways are basically static. T'ai chi is slightly different in this one point: It helps you to find a *moving* center. It's a movement meditation; you move your center with you. Although you are constantly in motion, you retain that quietness and stillness.

Experiment with this as you are sitting here now. I want you to physically find the place where you think your center is. Let your arms rest in your lap so you feel compact and balanced, sitting with a straight back. When you want to be quiet, just let your movement subside and diminish, and you will slowly come to a real stillness and centeredness. If you think you have to stop all movement, then you will become tense and rigid. You may look quiet from the outside, but inside there will be all kinds of tension and confusion. When you allow your movement to come to rest, you don't stop moving. Allow yourself to be like a pond that has been stirred up and slowly returns to a calm, smooth surface. Movement diminishes, but it's still there, like the stillness of this quiet pond, where there are still little ripples from time to time.

Now imagine that this is a zazen class and the master is watching you. You want to do a good job so you are really holding yourself very still. Now let's say you feel some discomfort in your back or somewhere else, and you feel a desire to move. The more you try to hold that position and deny that discomfort, the worse the discomfort becomes. Now let your body go a little and let movement happen. Instead of fighting it, let it happen and follow it. Let your spine sway a little from side to side. If you follow the movement, it will eventually curve around some way and return to your center.

If you think of a gentle uplift from the top of your head, then your spine will be quite straight without rigid holding. Let your spine be like a willow that moves with the wind, and then returns to straightness. Let all these curving movements get smaller and smaller. Eventually you will get to the point where you seem to be sitting still, but actually this movement is still circulating in your body. This is very comfortable and easy for your back, because you have allowed movement to come to rest instead of fighting it and becoming tense. You maintain the same kind of moving energy within your stillness.

As you're doing this, be aware of your breathing pattern. Try to breathe very fully, without forcing it. Sometimes we say "observing the breathing." This does not mean that you are outside of it; it means that you just follow it, and go with it. Don't force the stomach to come out, for instance, just because you think it should be healthier.

In t'ai chi, we call the breath-energy the ch'i. It is the energy that we use as we move. The lower abdomen just below the navel is called the tant'ien, and is considered to be both a reservoir for the ch'i, and the center from which our movement originates. Tan means the distilled vital essence, and also the rich, red color of blood. T'ien means field or place. So the tant'ien is the field of energy, the intrinsic energy, the reservoir of your vital force. The tant'ien corresponds to the Japanese hara or the sufi kath. Focusing attention on the breathing and the tant'ien is a useful way of becoming centered.

T'ai chi emphasizes a continuous circular breathing pattern. Circular means that you do not stop breathing out to breathe in, or the other way around. The letting go of your breath is the beginning of the coming in. This happens automatically when you just take a few minutes to do breathing. I emphasize this because it is very important that you realize the circular flow of your breathing. As you think of circular breathing, can you visualize the pattern of the relationship to your body? Is it a circle that goes running up the back and down the front of your torso? Do you visualize the air as an abstract pattern coming out of your nostrils, going down to the back part of your spine, coming back? How do you see it? Is it counterclockwise or clockwise? Does it turn horizontally or vertically, or does it go in a diagonal pattern? How is it? The circle expands, contracts, and changes. Make this circle a little more flexible. In t'ai chi movement, that circle goes all around. All the extensions of your body originate in your center, and then return to center again. You have all these individual loops and circles that keep coming back into this sphere of energy which is somewhere in your center. During the meditation process you allow that to happen. When all the imagery in your thoughts becomes your bodily feeling, then the first movement begins.

Now concentrate a little more into the base of your spine where you sit. If you're not sitting straight, try to sit straighter so you can really feel it. Breathe a little deeper and see if you can feel each disc of your back moving in relation to that expansion and contraction. Feel the back part of your spine with your breathing. Breathe a little bigger without tensing or forcing. See if you can identify that circular curve. If we had straight-backed chairs, it would be very good for you to feel your body leaning and pushing against it. The other day I had a belt on that was touching the back part of the wooden chair, and it kept saying "dat dat dat dat, dat .. dat .. dat .. dat, dat, dat-datdat"—as my back was going up and down with my breathing. That should happen in your back. Most of us have a certain part of our back that is not as flexible as it could be. When you feel the length, how does it curve back, and when does this happen?

Stretch a little longer—in length, in breadth, and in time. Don't think of holding your breath longer—think of extending that length of your spine longer each time. Space it longer if you can. Now can you also go sideways instead of just up? Can you let that circular feeling open outwards through your shoulder blades and out into your shoulders? It goes up and opens and fans out. See if you can get energy out through your shoulder blades, as far as your shoulders. It should affect your back, and the upper parts of your arms. Each time, keep returning to the beginning of the breathing circle.

T'ai chi has often been misunderstood by people observing it. They see a straight spine and ask, "How come your back is so stiff?" If your back is stiff, you are practicing t'ai chi incorrectly. This circular movement may not show so markedly, but your back must have the continuation of this flow. The next time you breathe way up, see if you can let the shoulder blades lift, and let the arms float forward and up just a little bit ... and then come down. As you expand, keep this flow moving out, and then when you recoil, just pull back into yourself. Let the movement begin in your chest and shoulders and flow out into your arms. Don't begin in your hands.

We are doing this sitting; it is slightly easier when you're standing. But standing and moving the legs properly is one of the most difficult things. The thigh usually hurts very much in the first few lessons of t'ai chi because of the tension of holding on. Sitting here, you don't have to worry about the legs.

Begin with the spine, and lift up in this breathing expansion. Your arms will begin lifting up at the shoulders and this lift will flow into your arms. Your

arms will lift slowly until they are almost horizontal.
You can think of a horizontal energy that keeps lifting
your arms until they are level and then goes out
through your fingertips. When your arms begin to sink
down, imagine that the space underneath your arms
is a soft, uneven supporting surface, like moving
water. Feel this surface moving slightly and supporting you as you balance on top of it. As your arms sink
down and come back in toward your body, allow the
upper part of the arm to come in first, and then pull
the rest back. Let the fingertips trail behind, as if
flowing behind the upper arm and shoulder. As you
settle, you will have the sense of sinking and the unity
of a flowing curve. Don't worry about watching the
length and height of your arm gesture, as long as it
has this flow action. And also don't take it literally
when I say level. It's like the water surface: It slants
and tips and curves when you move, but all of these
curves are only small departures from the straight
level line. So don't say, "I've got to stay completely
parallel." The whole idea is to *not* get limited.

Each time, you have to go through the whole sequence of this energy flow. It starts from way down
here in your tant'ien, up through your chest and
shoulders, and keeps expanding through and through
as your arms rise . . . until you feel the energy come
out of your fingertips and then the return happens.
This is why just the feeling of this first rise and fall
takes months and months to begin to learn in actual
t'ai chi practice. The problem is that it can become
very dull. You have nothing to hang on to. It's too
bland—all you do is raise your arm. All of us are
strong enough to raise our arms and put our arms
down. The challenge is not the flashiness of the movement; the challenge is to get the feeling of one thing
at a time—*now*. Each extension of the energy becomes that new moment. This is the most difficult
movement of t'ai chi. All the other motifs are really
just extensions of this first basic t'ai chi movement.

A good way to get the feeling of this movement
is in a hot bath or a swimming pool. The water will

support your arms more than the air because it has greater density. The next time you are in water, sit in a cross-legged position, and just let your spine float upward like grass, like water weeds flowing up. Then let your arms flow upwards, and let them rest on the substance of the water. Air also has its own density and space, and you can let the air around you support you in the same way.

This space around you is called yin space, in contrast to the yang space that is occupied by your body. I want you to feel your yang, physical self accepting the yin space—playing hide-and-seek with it. Be aware of the space around you as if it were water touching you. Look at me now, but look only at my outline, and the space around me. Let me disappear and see only the remaining movement in the air.

Now feel this yourself. Let your body disappear into the space/energy around you. You are resting on this space and being moved by it. There's nothing that you have to do or force. All your yang is settling, expanding, feeling. You enfold it all over, equally, smoothly. You feel like clouds, like steam, with its little tiny particles. You have a sense of almost getting lost within it, and then recapture an awareness of your own reality in that relationship. Both things are happening at the same time. In order to understand the yang, the solid, you must come to know the yin, the space around you. Learn to trust this energy and play with it.

Now as you are sitting here, just let your arms float up and then let the elbows sink down again. The entire movement is sequential. It really makes you go through all the parts of your body with this whole breathing/feeling process. Not one place is neglected. This is why t'ai chi is a healing exercise used to correct joint problems, or any other congestion or blockage that divides the body. When you practice t'ai chi, you become aware of where your body is stiff and divided, and you feel how you are misusing your body. You discover how your movement is fragmented, and you also learn how to move in a more flowing way so as to reconnect your movements into a smooth, easy sequence.

If you learn dancing or movement, people will say move your arms. In t'ai chi I would say here's a space being moved by your hands, or here are hands being moved by space. T'ai chi energy is in *in*action, by not doing. But when I say inaction in English it sounds like paralysis, instead of the happening that occurs when you stop doing things intentionally. With intention you think, "I have to do it," and usually "I don't want to," or "I'm afraid I can't," so you soon get into conflict. T'ai chi can bring you into a unity in which you don't think, and movement just happens. When you really allow yourself to give in and open up, your whole body tingles, your pores seem to open, you get goose bumps.

It's *both* the feeling of letting go *and* the feeling of awareness. It's not one-sided. I could put on some nice music and say, "OK, let's let go for a while, and pretty soon you will be relaxed." That's like providing you a big bathtub of pink bubbly champagne for you to submerge in and indulge in. That's only a one-sided way of doing it. T'ai chi doesn't allow you that kind of license to say, "OK, I'll just have a good time dancing." I want you to enjoy it, but at the same time I want you to be really aware of what you're doing. In t'ai chi, there's an outside and inside awareness together. It does not have that kind of introversion that so much meditation has.

Now try this same beginning arm-lift sequence while standing. As the arms come down, let your legs go into the flow. Imagine that you are standing on water, and let your base become soft and yielding. You see, I ask you to think of the yin space as if it were more solid, and to think of the yang space as if it were more transparent. This is a readjustment of space which you can work with wherever you are. Think of your feet extending beneath the floor. Sometimes we use the imagery of having roots spreading down into the ground. It's as if the sole of your foot is really testing where you're standing, and you feel this from your center.

Now close your eyes for a minute and let your body go slightly lopsided. Don't worry about falling. Shift your weight from one leg to another. Be insecure at first, and then just go with the movement of this imbalance. Just keep going with the curve and it will eventually find its way back to center. The circle gets smaller and smaller, and you get closer and closer to yourself as you settle down. You have to do this with resilience in your legs—without tightening your knees, without pulling your thigh muscles, without blocking your calf muscles. Let your joints flow, and just sort of roll and rock around. Imagine that you're in the middle of a wave.

I spoke to three surfing champions from Hawaii who watched the t'ai chi group working and they said, "Hey! that's interesting—this is exactly what we have been working on. We have developed a surfing yoga and that's exactly what we're doing." Those of you who have done surfing, you *know*. How can you stay on the surfboard without constantly letting the body give with the wave? Try this while standing on a waterbed, and then walk on it. It's something you cannot fight: You must *give in* to it and *then* you can begin.

You have to have the patience and willingness to give in before the real sense of the imagery comes through. The difficult part of t'ai chi practice is how long can you sway around and keep doing this first arm-lifting movement before you get bored and want to go on to some other movement? How do you stay with it? If you begin to think this is too slow and is not working for you, just imagine doing zazen in a zendo. This is like flying compared to zazen where you just sit in lotus position with your back straight. Even zazen is not really a solid-set stillness; it's really a moving stillness. You are breathing and you feel that marvelous thin line flowing upward and that settling back down into center. You are moving into stillness.

Now let's experiment with this movement in a somewhat different way. As you sway around, move your arms a little from your shoulders and rotate your torso from right to left and back. Let your arms swing freely and flop against your body. Notice how the shoulder swing affects your base. Do a swing, and then just before the end of the swing, begin to rotate back in the other direction. Rotate and swing out until you feel the pull in your arms, and then slow down. This swing really helps you to sense how the movement of the upper body is connected through the spine and down into the pelvis.

When you pull back, see if you can feel the back settling down, pulling the arms back sequentially, with the fingertips last. Swing into it, and pull back. As you swing out, your body is slightly lopsided. When you pull back, find the middle and then let the arms flow out to the other side so you can feel the sense of the circle. As you do this swinging, you will find that your weight shifts on your feet. As you swing to the right, most of your weight comes off your left foot. Actually pick up this unweighted foot, and then let it down again as you swing back. Each time you give in to a new base.

So far, we are still keeping the pelvic area pretty steady. Allow some movement in the hip joints and thighs. If you pivot from side to side, you feel that your spine rotates with this movement. You have to make adjustment with your whole foot, keeping contact with the floor so you don't feel unsteady.

Now let's use these ideas in the movement called Embracing the Moon, or carrying the t'ai chi sphere. Imagine that you are carrying a soapy, slippery sphere about the size of a basketball in your hands. Play with holding this slippery ball and tip it around. If you hold it too tightly, it will slip away, and if you hold it too loosely, it will fall. As you move it around, your balance will change and you will have to shift your base. Make adjustments with your base without thinking which foot you have to move. Get into the feeling of the imagery. Give the sphere weight if you need to. Pantomime, and imagine that you're holding something very heavy.

As you shift around, your weight has to be adjusted on your legs. Do this without thinking which foot must move next. Curve out, and move back in a loop. It's not "Go there—and then come back." It is the whole circle: Loop, and back, and loop again. It's a circle that you can feel within: In relationship to your legs, in relationship of one arm to another, in relationship with the floor. Continue to just play with this sphere a little longer.

Now let this sphere slowly increase in size until the whole front of your body contacts the surface of this soapy sphere. Continue to move with the sphere touching the inside of your arms and the front of your torso and legs. The whole t'ai chi movement starts with the simple understanding that your body is the center of your energy sphere. Your body, with awareness of its different parts, all comes together as a center in moving circular motion. All the different movements of the t'ai chi ch-uan are variations of this flowing circular movement. Sometimes it is a small circle, sometimes it is large, sometimes the circle becomes a long elliptical curve, returning back in a double loop like a figure eight.

If you play with variations of this t'ai chi sphere, you can discover for yourself all the movements that are part of the form. You discover how all these variations have the same kind of flow, and how each movement continues easily into another.

I don't want to show you the form of t'ai chi ch'uan too early, because you will probably only see the structure, which will confuse you. You will only build up more tension, trying too hard to control and imitate the shape. You have to work through the feeling of your body gradually, allowing the form to emerge and become you. T'ai chi is an art: not to be taught, but to be experienced. You can always learn a form later, after you get into this circular flow. Each teacher has a slightly different form, a slightly different way of doing t'ai chi. You don't have to believe me or any master. Your own practice will tell you what feels right to you. I want to show you how much pleasure I can derive from what I do, and how I understand and remind myself about the essence of t'ai chi.

I learned many many forms of t'ai chi when I was a child. We were moving from one village to another, running away from the Japanese-Chinese war. In each village there was someone who did t'ai chi, and I did t'ai chi with him. As a child I didn't concern myself with whether he was the "best" master, or whether he was famous, or would give me a certificate. I just did it with whoever was there. Any form is only *one* expression of the essence of t'ai chi, so don't get stuck with only one part of the whole. If you limit yourself to the structure of any one form you will lose the essence.

Later I will gradually show you some short sequences and motifs, which will give you a structure to work on, something to practice. When you come out and practice with me tomorrow begin with awareness of movement outside and movement inside your body. Use the ocean, use the wind blowing, become aware of your breathing. See if you can begin to move *from the sense of where you are*. Follow that beginning of energy and go with it.

Now let me just see you try to begin. Let your body settle into your base. Then sway a little, and discover where you are. Make adjustments of your feet, and then get together and centered. At the same time, don't plant your feet down. The minute you try to say, "This is a nice spot to hang onto" you are stuck, like a nail. You must feel the movement underneath your feet, as if you are walking on the ocean. Feel this lift of energy through the expansion of your breath and the extension of your body happening together. Then work towards the lift of the arms from your back and shoulder. When the arms lift up, let them rest on a surface that is uneven and moves like the waves of the ocean.

When you get the feeling of this flow, play with

the t'ai chi sphere. Use the inside of your hands and arms to form the shape of the sphere and then begin to move it around. Keep the sense of the sphere as you play with it and let it change slowly. Let it grow large or shrink small. You may extend one side of the sphere into a longer curve as if the sphere became a long egg-shape. You may bring it sideways, making it a little lower. You may lift it up a little higher, or let it move around you. Be sure to always bring this curve back in so you don't lose contact with your center.

Keep your spine in the middle, so you always have a place to return to. This is like in kundalini yoga, the serpent, that fire energy that keeps moving in your spine. That feeling of one spinal disc at a time keeps moving and falling in a circle, so you know where your center is. If you bend your back, if you move your center, then you don't know where to return. You have to keep that upright torso as a reference point.

You have to maintain a sense of your center as you do this free-form moving with the sphere. Keeping centered means that you realize that this particular arm movement is related to your center *this* way. That particular leg opening out that way is related back to your center, *this* way. So you have something to retain as you move. That's to keep you from bathing in your pink, bubbly champagne bath and just having a good, lazy time—you may become so relaxed that you feel immobile, and pretty soon you fall asleep. T'ai chi should awaken you; you keep this centeredness and connection with your surroundings.

Do you see everybody around you? Do you see the chairs, do you see the floor, do you see the person next to you? Keep your ears open, too. Do you hear the feet shuffling? Do you hear the talking in the next room? Do you hear your own breathing and the person's breathing next to you? Keep that alertness open all around, without losing your center. This is the t'ai chi meditation. If you do it this way, then the form will continue to challenge you; it will become spontaneous with the human body movement as you go through the process. It's very easy to begin, if you *let* it begin that way. It's very difficult to stay with; it's so easy to get lost. That's why we have the form.

Early morning, before breakfast, is a really good time to do t'ai chi. As you begin, you can do deep breathing and then extend that breathing into movement. Every time you begin, you have to recapture that center all over again. Even after you practice quite a bit, there's no safe place where you know "I can always begin there." You can't depend on past experiences or an accumulation of them. You always begin right here, where you are, with your sense of yourself and your surroundings now.

My ideal of this workshop is that in some way we can recreate that process of the old masters who created the original t'ai chi. How did they do it? If you can experience one part of this original individual creation, maybe something will come out of *you*. Then the t'ai chi is yours. It's *your* t'ai chi ch'uan.

II

Whatever I say to you is either a repetition, a reaffirmation, or a new attempt at this moment to relate to you what I'm trying to do. It's a new experience each time. I want to sense what you begin to feel, and what part of you wants to work now. I'm not always right: Sometimes I tune in with a couple of you and leave the rest of you out. Certain things mean more to one body than another. But in a week's time, we'll do many things, and somehow I'll get to all of you.

All these things we are doing illustrate one main point: The continuity of letting one movement lead smoothly into another without any breaks, hesitations, or sudden changes. But how can we bring about this coordination in the body? There's no use to follow the whole sequence of t'ai chi ch'uan and imitate all the motions. If I saw everybody go out on the deck and do it in unison, I wouldn't say "Bravo!" I would say "How sad." So many people just go through the motions mechanically and that's the end of true creativity. I would be unhappy to see that happening to t'ai chi movement. T'ai chi may look from the outside like a pattern or structure, but what is happening inside the body must be very different. T'ai is neither a set structure nor chaos. Not this. Not that. It is a different kind of organization which cannot be known by learning a set of patterned movements.

This is why I told you in the beginning that I'm

not going to give you forms immediately. This relieves some of your anxiety because you don't have to worry about copying or repeating the movements exactly. I could teach you like some teachers who begin with details and stances. "OK. Let's begin from the beginning. Here is position one. OK. And you say, 'How far should I raise my arms?' About here. OK. It's too high. Lower them two inches. Part two: You turn your right wrist 90° and move to the right. Now move the left hand over the right, and move your foot exactly 45° to your right. You put your toe down, lift your heel and touch."

This kind of teaching seems to me like putting on another straight-jacket. Always you are worrying about what to do next, always thinking. You do too much thinking already, and this thinking always interferes with the flow of your movement. You don't have to prove to yourself or anybody else that by the end of the week you have learned a certain amount. The minute that you have a goal, you keep thinking about that, and then you're really not doing what's happening here.

Many people learn t'ai chi just so they can show it off to somebody else. They learn certain movements from the outside, but they miss the inside, the essence. And some t'ai chi teachers also have made this mistake. I can't identify with a lot that I hear about t'ai chi. When people come to me and talk about t'ai chi, I often have this double reaction. Either I have to just keep listening to them until I find some common ground with them, or I may have to go the other way —maybe I'll have to say I'm *not* a t'ai chi teacher. I have already eliminated the word ch'uan from t'ai chi ch'uan for this one reason. The ch'uan is the form. It means literally "a fist," a hand, the art of fighting. T'ai chi ch'uan means "The movement phrase that is used for defense, for practice of your body/mind, based on the idea of t'ai chi." T'ai chi itself is a much more open, inclusive term.

T'ai chi is also a meditation. Meditation does not require isolation. You can meditate now. We are meditating if we really hear each other speaking, if you hear what you are saying yourself and hear the pounding of the surf out there. I hear you, I sense you here, and this awareness process is meditation. This process quiets you down and opens you up. Sometimes you have to make a special point to meditate more immediately, more effectively, because of your need. If you really have a very hectic day with things pulling you all over and unbalancing you, then at times it is useful to retreat temporarily in order to return to your center faster. You meditate, you try to give in and receive what is happening within you and around you.

At other times it might be much more useful to shout and move. I remember working as an architectural draftsman one summer in a big office building. I was in a glass cubicle with the boss observing every move I made. I used to go to the bathroom as often as I could, and when nobody else was there I would scream and dance and swing and jump up and down. Then I would feel much better and I could come back and work for a while. I also used to ask to be the errand boy when something had to be delivered to another building so that I could walk and move.

T'ai chi shows that there is no such thing as absoluteness. When you accept this, then you begin. T'ai chi is the experience you have as you are searching. People say, "I am searching for truth." Intellectually you are searching for truth, but what is truth, what is wisdom? *Wisdom is that particular emergence from your own spontaneity of an identification with what you know of the universe around you.*

Most of the time, we move. Now you notice, watching me, I'm not talking without any movement. In fact, I move a lot. I'm a moving person; I have a lot of energy that has to be expressed. I'm a very energetic person, and I throw myself around a lot if I don't practice t'ai chi. There is nothing wrong with throwing yourself around, nothing wrong with that other side of the energy which is the same as calmness.

The minute you use two words, there seem to be two different things. He's moving; he's quiet. T'ai chi integrates these two extremes. When you meditate, you realize you're moving and being quiet at the same time. Your energy is furiously moving, extending, feeling, while your physical self is settling down quietly. Watch a potter centering the clay on the potter's wheel. You see that furious motion of the turning—yet the clay seems not to move; it doesn't budge because it is centered. It's right there, as if it's standing still. Potting is clearly a zen art.

Zen, or ch'an in Chinese, means "solitary person's heart and mind opening to awareness of the sign from heaven." T'ai chi is zen, is dhyana, is meditation, is yoga. These are all different terms for the same kind of path, the same way of being. The only way you can identify your *own* feeling of what yoga, or zen, or dhyana, or t'ai chi is all about is through your own experience. It's there. You don't have to put it into words.

T'ai chi has a particular flow pattern. But if you pick up a t'ai chi book, usually it has a series of poses and a lot of little footprints in the directions. It reminds me of Arthur Murray's old dance manuals with footprints on the floor, for doing cha-cha-cha and tango. People never could learn to dance through the Arthur Murray dance books, so finally they had to pay their fee to go to the dance school. You cannot learn movement that way, because you try to fit yourself into that rigid, fragmented pattern. Because of teaching problems, most masters count the sequence of t'ai chi ch'uan in numbers. "This is movement one; this is movement two." Basically, this is all wrong, and I've been trying to teach t'ai chi somewhat differently.

T'ai chi is a very simple movement pattern. You play with your base and you begin to discover all the variations of the movement; then you allow that circular flow to take you in different directions, and then you revolve, and finally you come back almost to the original spot where you began. This is an important point: T'ai chi must help you to come all the way around. It's that cycle, that journey that takes you and somehow brings you back again—without saying, "forty-five degrees that way, two steps forward, etc." So right away you know all your anxiety of trying to get somewhere is futile. Why do you want to get somewhere? You come back to the same place anyway! We all smile because we know this is true.

You come here for a week; you pay quite a bit for the facility, and for some of my fee. This is money you could have used for a lot of other things, but you make a sacrifice to come. You want to get something to take with you. And you *will* retain something, in spite of yourself. But if you keep trying too hard, you will get in your own way. I teach dance, and sometimes I see a student writing notes like mad. "What do you do with those notes?" He says, "Well, when I go back and teach my students I forget, so I have to take notes." I say, "Why don't you spend time in practice so you can *do* it? The notes will not help you to *do* it when you go back." There are many, many people who want to rely on something which is really behind them or in front of them, not *now*. T'ai chi is now, the same as gestalt therapy, the same as a lot of techniques that stress immediacy, and immediate response, so you can really dig into what's happening at this given moment.

I would like to try one thing with you now. Pair up and face each other. Sit cross-legged so you're close enough to each other to be comfortable. I would like you to hook your right arms and hook your right hands together. This is a double helix which gives a nice close-fit feeling without strain. Cup your left hand under your right elbow so that your elbow stays relaxed. Take some time just to get into the feeling of your touch: Feel the warmth and the texture of the contact. See each other and try to blend the looking with the physical connection between you.

Go beyond the distinction of the particular structure of the face, the forehead, the color of the eyes, the nose, the mouth—look at the total feeling of it, instead of particular details. See if you can get a feeling of the whole look. Take it in until it's not a strange

face; it's a face that you really know, that really reflects you. You can do this same experiment alone with
a mirror.

Check your shoulder tension, check the grasp of
your hand. Feel the inside of your hand—there are
another person's fingers. They are there moving a little
bit, and you must allow that movement to be. At the
same time there is some feeling of the other person's
energy coming through there from his body. Make a
circular connection through seeing and listening and
touching. If you feel like blinking, go ahead and blink
—don't try to keep your eyes open.

Now check to see if you are breathing easily.
Maybe you could let go a little more and breathe a
little more so that your shoulder and forearm become
more free. See if you can feel each other's breathing
through the hand and arm connection. Can you feel
the gentle heaving of your torso? Do your thighs
move a little when you breathe? Are you connecting
in a very easy, relaxed way?

Sometimes I use the image of a flower in a mirror.
Let's contemplate that image. Whatever passes by the
mirror is reflected impartially, and when it goes past
the mirror, the mirror does not retain any image.
There's no way of retaining or saving anything. You
don't have to worry about leaving your mark on the
mirror. The mirror image illustrates that mirror-mind,
that emptiness that can take in whatever is there. If
you simply reflect the other person as what he is or
what she is, there's no prejudice, there's no way of
seeing anything that could create self-consciousness.
It's just a clear reflection. When somebody looks at
you, you should allow that openness. There is no need
to feel uncomfortable being observed.

We could also use the metaphor of the moon coming out and casting its image on the surface of calm
water. When the moon goes behind the cloud, we
don't see it any more. When the breeze comes and
the water ripples and flows, we may see many, many
distorted moons. But it's not the water's intention to
reflect or to disturb the image. Water and moon and

breeze and cloud are individual separate entities flowing, existing together as one, without any demand or need to say, "You must do this for me; I must do that for you."

Now lift your hand up and pull each other a little bit and feel this opposition. Extend your arms enough so that you feel that your whole arms are free to move. Now join your left arms in the same way. It's a very crossed feeling. I want you to unwind and untangle as you move, without releasing your hands. This gives you a new dimension. It's like the two arms of a churning machine. You will have a feeling of being pulled and twisted around, but yet it's very centered and balanced.

Even within this restricted sitting position there is quite a wide range of movement possible. There's a folk dance in which the partners keep their hands joined throughout a long sequence of turning, twisting, and unwinding.

Now see if you can relax that grip; keep only a very slight touch, and continue to move. Discover your wrists and how they rotate. Now slow down a bit. Let your torso also move with the movement of your arms. Let your body rock on top of your base a little.

If you are holding your muscles in tension, your arms will be getting tired. Let go. This is a good time to talk about manipulation. When you begin working on a form, first you follow it, and then you begin to repeat it. The minute you think you've got it, then you begin to manipulate it with your preconceptions. This is why t'ai chi works so slowly. If you stay with that slow, now, happening, you don't have to remember if you have finished half a turn or half a curve, so you do not have the anxiety of thinking, "I must finish it in a circle." You are always there in the moment, and you let it happen.

Now as we're still sitting here, let's do the motif called the Cloudhand, or moving your hands like clouds. Let go of your partner's hands and move away from him.

The Cloudhand is basically a movement that stirs up your tant'ien energy upward and outward and then circles back. If we cut an apple in half, we see two smaller circles overlapping in the center. Your spine is like the core and your arm motion is like the two overlapping circles.

Each hand, in turn, scoops up energy from the tant'ien and rises up the center line of your chest before turning outward, revolving, sinking downward, and curving back to the tant'ien. Then the other hand picks up the motion of the first and goes through the same cycle. Your torso pivots to follow the hand as it turns and revolves outward and downward.

As you do this, think of using your body in a functional way. Scoop up space as you lift your hand. As you begin to turn, let the space spill out and run downward like water. Then your shoulder and elbow get heavy, and as your elbow sinks, the hand trails behind the elbow and rotates. The hand revolves to face outward and downward in a slow stroking motion that circles back to the tant'ien and comes to rest as the other hand picks up the movement.

Vary the range and the scope of the movement. Try turning only a little, and then as far as you can easily turn. Do it large and small, high and low. Let your hands float all over and around you. Explore all the possibilities contained within this simple movement. As long as the movement flows easily and continuously as you curve and rotate, you are fine. As you continue your practice, all these many different movements will gradually condense into what is called moving hands like clouds—that beautiful rotation resolving into another beginning, followed by another rotation resolving into yet another beginning.

If you understand the *principles* of the movement, you will not get stuck in worrying about the irrelevant *details*—how large it should be, or exactly when to begin turning, etc. If you only pay attention to details, you will feel awkward and confined. The minute you feel confined and you stop to think, then the flow gets stagnant and polluted. Pretty soon your movement becomes dead and looks as if you are only trying to copy the master's instructions. If there is any rule in the learning process of t'ai chi, it's the minute that you feel confined into anything, get out of it first, and then flow back into the form once more.

Now let's stand up and work on the feeling of the base and legs, and then we'll combine this with the Cloudhand. First just get in touch with the feeling of your legs under you. Your knees should be slightly bent so that you settle down toward the earth more. Now walk around slowly and turn your body as you walk. T'ai chi teaches you not to transfer your weight too suddenly, and to always keep your base between your legs. There are a few movements in t'ai chi that require you to stand on one leg, but basically your weight stays centered between your legs, ready to move in any direction. You always use the easiest, most efficient way of carrying your weight. Whether you spread your legs wide or bring them close together, your base should always be between them.

Now slow down your steps as you continue to move and turn, and focus your awareness on the feeling in your feet. Do they clunk down like bricks, or do they reach down to the ground? Often you see t'ai chi practiced with the heel always touching first. The reason for that is to help you to really roll the foot down slowly using one part at a time, so that you can thoroughly feel your contact with the ground. You use the whole bottoms of your feet and make them soft and resilient. Rolling your heel down first is a good way to glide into it and still keep your weight in the middle. The whole foot, including the toe, should grasp the ground with an intimate, sensitive contact as if it were a hand. You don't touch the ground by just tapping with your heel and pointing with your toes. You don't ignore or resist or fight the ground; you welcome it and sink into it.

Imagine that you are on unsafe ground. There are thorns sticking up here and there, so that if you just clunk your foot down and put all your weight on it, you're going to get stabbed. Some of the ground is slippery and small rocks may make your feet roll out from under you. You're always feeling and sensing, and always ready to change and adjust. You should feel that you are carrying your weight in the middle, in the region of your pelvis. If you feel that you are carrying your weight only on the ball of the foot, then you will move differently and your leg will get tired. Your feet and legs should have a sense of taking in and feeling the ground. This is why primitive dancing and oriental dancing often has a low stance and a sense of really liking the ground. This kind of movement is much more human and naturally aware of its connection with the earth. This is the opposite of most ballet dancing in which the dancer tries to touch the ground as little as possible for a theatrical and ethereal effect.

Now think of your base as if your legs are just part of a flexible pedestal, or an amoeba-like tree trunk that goes out to the ground in all directions from your body. Your weight is being carried on all sides, not just on your legs or in front; the back and sides are just as important. When you move in this way you very rarely get yourself cross-legged or unstable.

What we're doing is to reacquaint ourselves with something that is very basic, like breathing, that we normally don't have to worry about. People who have respiratory diseases often have to go to a clinic and spend hours to re-learn how to breathe properly. When we find that our bodies are not moving as naturally as they could, then we have to take time to re-learn the natural way, the easy way of moving functionally. This kind of practice should happen all the time. T'ai chi needs to be practiced daily in your own movements; it's not something separate that you do only in the morning.

As you move around now, be aware of the space between you and other people and objects. Your awareness of this space and others' movements should affect you somehow, and modify your movement. You turn and move differently when you are related to the space and the objects and the movements around you through your awareness and responses to them. If you walk by a window, you may slow down as you look outside. If you move into an open space you may extend your arm farther. You are experiencing the changing events around you, and also the constant feeling in your own center as you move and respond. T'ai chi is the awareness of the constancy within all this change. Your awareness of what you are doing, and how you are responding and opening up to outside events develops into a whole, more fully complete movement than what you alone can do.

When you feel natural and comfortable simply moving around with a good solid base, try pivoting and turning and continue to move in gentle curves. Now incorporate the Cloudhand arm movement with your turning and stepping. In the t'ai chi ch'uan, the Cloudhand travels only to the left. When I play with the form, I reverse it and go to the right as well. It's a very nice feeling and I don't feel so lopsided.

Once you get into the feel of the rotation and revolution you can just allow the energy of the movement to carry you as far or as little as it wants to go. Most teachers ask you to do the Cloudhand as a very small subtle gesture. I like you to try it large. I want you to feel the connection through your whole body. After you get the feeling of this big movement, then you can let it slowly diminish in size and still keep the flow as the gesture becomes more subtle.

I have a friend who took a film of an old master in Taiwan by the ocean. It's very beautiful. I may be able to do more fancy things—I have certain skills and a strong body—but that old man has a subtlety, with so many more years of practice, that I can't possibly match. So right away, there's no comparison. There's no way of saying, "Your way is better than mine." There's no such thing.

The form slowly crystallizes and settles into what you know. After many years of practicing, when you really know t'ai chi and you have done so many curves with your arms, you will be able to do a gentle crystallized small curve and make it look like ten million

large waves going around. You will have discovered
the simplicity of the curve in your body. But if your
master, after sixty years of experiencing the form,
does a simple flick of the wrist and says, "You do that.
Turn, flip, do that. Keep doing this"—that is super-
imposing upon you that sixty years of doing large
circles that developed into this tiny little form which
looks so exquisite. Unfortunately you can only put it
on the shelf and admire it; it can never become you
that directly. You can only do the circle for years until it becomes smaller and smaller and more crystallized—until finally this flick of a wrist becomes that
beautiful circle for you. That's the reason for my approach to doing t'ai chi: to really get into the feeling
of it and at the same time realize that you're at the
periphery of the form.

When you practice, you are there in the focal
center. You can go either this way or that way as you
please. When you are most centered, you can feel both
directions of the circle simultaneously. So when you
do Cloudhand, think of extending your curve one way
with one hand, and then carrying on to the turning
curve. When you have your base a little wider, you
can shift your weight more easily.

I like to let the center of my palm rise about level
with my eyes, so that I can easily watch the rotation
of the hand. If you look at your hand as you move,
you won't get dizzy and you'll have a better sense of
where your center is. As the view behind the hand
goes swinging from the ocean to trees, to sunlight, to
railing, to somebody's feet, many pairs of legs, each is
just part of the chain. The constant is where you are
looking at your hand. Don't lift your elbows—let your
elbow move down, droop down. Feel the inside of
your arm coming toward you as your hand sinks down.

Use the image of an eye inside your palm looking
at you and then panning out as your palm turns, looking all around and then looking down to the ground.
Your hand is going through a cyclical change. If you
listen to the ocean, the waves, it's not broken and
staccato. It has one long flow of a wave as it lifts,

reaches the heights, and subsides. Your arm is also moving just like the sound of the ocean. It has its lift, the height of the wave, and then the downward flow until it becomes settled. Don't let your arms go too far away from your body. As you move you must feel the space between your arms and your body so that you don't lose awareness of how they are related.

Another important thing is to let the body sink as the hand rises at the beginning of the movement, and let the body rise as the hand pushes down. The t'ai chi literature talks about "the rise and fall." The minute I try to explain things like this in English, I run out of words. There are ten different ways of thinking of the rising and falling in Chinese. Now you think of rising—is it active lifting? There's a different word, lifting, and its opposite might be pulling down. T'ai chi helps us to find the subtlety, the different ways of finding that one gesture. You get a three-dimensional, many-faceted way of saying that one thing so clearly and so simply. The purity of t'ai chi is that you can play with all these different ways of saying it—if you have to say it in words—and then you crystallize it by practicing the movement with the feeling. The movement can have everything in it. It can have the rise and fall, the lift and the sinking down—and all the other things at the same time.

Next I want to work again with the t'ai chi sphere, and then with the movements that immediately follow the beginning arm lift in the long form of t'ai chi ch'uan. These early movements are slight variations of the t'ai chi sphere. Stay with the feeling of the base and the movement of the legs that we have been working on, and imagine that you are carrying a large soap bubble. I want you to feel the fragile, resilient, elusive surface of this soap bubble in your hands.

Carry this sphere of energy fairly low, about the level of your navel, as if it were quite heavy. This will help you to feel the connection of your upper body with your base, and help you to sink down a little and get your base underneath this sphere. As you turn to the right, step out to the right in order to keep your base solidly under your movements. Feel how the weight of this imaginary sphere is transmitted down through your body to your base. As you do this, keep your spine straight by imagining that it rises and floats up from the pelvis in a gentle uplift. It shouldn't be rigid and tight.

Let your hands move freely all around the surface of the sphere, so that you hold it with a flowing, changing contact. Let the energy-bubble slowly become smaller until your hands are close together as if you are holding a small creature, or sheltering a tiny robin's egg that is ready to hatch. Let this energy move inside your hands without clenching or crushing it. Nurture it and be very tender and gentle. Now let this energy expand as if it were a growing thing, gradually pushing your hands apart. As this sphere of energy grows larger, it also contacts the insides of your forearms. As it grows even larger, pushing your hands and arms apart, it contacts your chest and torso as well. Eventually, you are embracing this huge sphere with your whole body, and you really have to settle down and dig into your base to support it.

As you continue to move with this sphere, let it take over, and just follow it as it moves and changes in size. If you think and decide how to move next, then your movements will be stiff and disjointed. But if you allow your thinking and feeling to circle into the sphere, then it has a way of moving by itself, and all you do is follow it. The sphere will take over and direct you and move you according to the movement that you have created and allowed within yourself. When you really give in to it, there is a great relief of responsibility and a freedom from judging yourself. You can't be wrong if you're not doing it, and the movement can't be wrong if you're just following.

Now let's go back to the beginning movement that we have already done. Stand easily and pay attention to your breathing. Allow the energy of your breathing to flow into your shoulders and your arms. They must lift slowly and sequentially from the shoulders, with the fingertips rising last. As your arms become level, let your elbows pull in and sink slowly as the rest of your arm follows. Settle down into your base a little as your arms sink down in front of you. Just take your time and allow it all to happen.

If you rush to finish this movement and say, "OK, I'm done. What next?" then the next movement would be arbitrary. But if you let the sinking energy of your arms curve to one side and become a sphere that moves, then you will find yourself turning spontaneously without having to think about it.

As you turn to the right, your right hand will scoop under to support the bottom of the sphere and begin to move out to the right while your left hand is above and slightly behind. Use the image of Grasping the Sparrow's Tail. It's as if your right hand is a sparrow flying to the right in slow motion while the left hand is following just above and behind it, trying to catch it.

If you keep trying to catch something that is very fast, you won't catch it. But if you make it move very slowly, if you just slow down and don't worry about catching, then the energy you want to catch comes around and catches you. As you turn far to the right, your hands revolve and change places as the movement loops around and moves back to the left again.

This slow pursuit around a sphere develops a moving circular relationship between the two hands. At any moment the two hands are on opposite points of the sphere. This movement is the essence of t'ai chi, in which the energy is very concentrated. All the different motifs are variations of this movement on the surface of a sphere. Each motif is a specific, clear actualization of this basic movement. Through the practice of the different motifs, you get a feel of the flow in your body that slowly crystallizes back again into this small, simple, concentrated spherical movement called Grasping the Sparrow's Tail.

The next sequence, called pung-lü-chi-an is one of the key motifs to illustrate how the specific movements grow and develop out of the concentrated spherical movement. Your hands revolve again and open up to about the size of a basketball, and you begin to turn back to the right. This is the beginning of the pung, or Embracing the Moon. Keep your base under you as you move. As you turn far to the right, your hands again revolve and begin to move back to the left in a widening horizontal circle that dips past tant'ien and curves up to shoulder level. This is called the lü. A rough translation of lü is "fitting into the shape." Sometimes we use this word for fitting into shoes or fitting into a form. As you turn to the left you have to settle down to receive the energy, which curves back in toward you and down a little.

Now the fingers of your left hand touch your right wrist as if you are feeling your pulse, and begin to push out and back to the right. This is called the chi, which means "leaning by squeezing." Although it is spelled the same, this chi is different from the chi of t'ai chi. There are many ways to do this. Some people push with the fingers, while some use the palm. Sometimes they touch the hand or the arm instead of the wrist. Later you can simply suggest the pushing, without touching. I like the feeling of touching the pulse so that I can really feel the circulation going through the wrist. The transition from moving to the left to pushing out to the right must be a smooth curve.

As you push with the left hand, the energy inside the circle of your arms increases and expands and pushes your arms open. Don't just detach your fingers, but see if you can feel the energy inside of the arms become so great that it literally pushes your arms open. You don't know exactly when that release will happen. It happens on its own because of your understanding of the energy inside of your arms swelling open. Try pushing very hard, so that you feel your arms trembling. Now look down into this space inside the circle of your arms right in front of you and feel the energy inside. I'm telling you to push hard in order to feel the energy. Usually, of course, you don't push with so much force.

As this circle of energy pushes your arms open, it

becomes bigger and bigger until it expands to include the circle of the group. As this circle continues to expand and move to the right, it goes beyond us and includes that whole mountain back there. Then it gets bigger and includes the whole continent and the ocean on the other side. If you can really feel this expansion, then your t'ai chi will have power in the very nice sense of the word. Power is not brute force; it's the essence of the vastness of your identification with the universal energy.

As this energy opens up and becomes enormous, it threatens you. What can you do with it? You can embrace it and gather it all back into your tant'ien. Receive this energy by letting your elbows drop and your palms turn up as you pull it back into your base. Don't lean back; if you do, the energy will push you over. Settle down and take it in as if you are catching a heavy object.

After you have gathered in all this energy, push it out again low from your tant'ien as if you are pushing a wall or something heavy. This is the beginning of the movement called the an. Push this energy way out to the edge of the horizon and let it curve back around to your left. Keep your elbows relaxed and slightly bent. If you stretch your arms too much you will become unbalanced. This contact with the energy on the far horizon becomes both a reaching and a receiving. The energy curves back to you and returns low, so you have to settle a little to gather it in beneath your feet and lift it into your tant'ien again.

Whenever you send energy out, you bring it back in again. It's like casting out a fish net and then drawing it back in. You send it out and then follow the curve and return. As this energy returns to you, you sink down to receive it into your center, and then you can send the energy out again. Unless you can really feel this energy process in your body, the movement will look very dry and very short.

Using images will help you to really feel this energy in your body. When you push out, imagine that you are pushing something very heavy and your body will tend to move in a vital way that is appropriate to that function. Then your beautiful t'ai chi movement will always have the potential of becoming a really energetic pushing when you need it. As you send energy way out to the horizon, imagine that you are sending a kite high into the sky. The higher the kite soars, the more you must be in touch with the pulling force in the string, and transmit this down into your tant'ien.

This pushing movement is also a sending out. Imagine that this energy is shooting out of the palms of your hands. If you go to Chinatown, you will see movie theaters with pictures of swordsmen, people flying, kung-fu combats, and sword-fights. These movies are corny and very bloody. The hero will hold his palm out, Fssssss—and daggers will come out of his palm, and then he will fly through the air. All this is fantasy, but it's based on taoist themes, and it is usually connected somehow with a taoist monk sitting in the mountains, practicing the ch'i. When I was a kid and had problems at home or got scolded, I used to wish that I could go to the mountains and study with the taoist monks. Instead I would go to the movies and come home feeling all that ch'i—my own identification with the fantasy of the daggers and flying. It's like your fantasies of Superman or the Green Hornet or Captain Marvel.

I want you to do t'ai chi as children would do it. Don't be so intellectual. You know the intellectual part of it. But the important thing is the discovery. Kids love it. I teach t'ai chi quite differently for children: We just have fun. They *love* this feeling of daggers coming out of their palms and they grunt like mad when they push.

When you send energy out, let it come back to you like a boomerang. Don't let it get lost out there. Gather it all into your tant'ien with your torso centered, and sink into your base to give you stability and contact with the ground. Then when you send this energy out again, you are sending from the base of your spine. As you reach, don't let the energy stop:

You keep curving and pull it back in again. Watch your fingertips and see if you can allow that energy and movement to continue smoothly.

It is very difficult to keep the energy flowing. You can't check, and you don't know how you're doing it wrong. When I was learning, my master would say, "No. Do it again." So I would do it again and he would say, "Now do it again, just do it again." You simply have to work with the movement until you discover it in your own body. I can show you how I do it, and I can give you some ideas about how it can be, but you have to discover it for yourself as you do it.

At breakfast we were talking about the Alexander method of working with the body, which has many similarities with t'ai chi. Before he developed his methods, Alexander used to lecture, but he got laryngitis all the time. So he looked at himself in a full-length mirror as he talked, to discover exactly how he was misusing his body. That's how he began to work out ways of discovering the tension and tightness that caused his laryngitis and other problems. It's very revealing, because so many illnesses show themselves in awkwardness and mis-coordination. We're all built the same, we all have the same kind of body structure. Some of you are a little stronger and more flexible but still the general shape of our t'ai chi movement is similar unless it's distorted by tension.

This is why I keep telling you not to use your muscles as if you are holding onto something rigidly. If you always use your body as if it is resting or moving, then you won't get tense and rigid. One of the main problems is tension in the shoulders and in the muscles of your neck, caused by holding your arms and sticking your chin out. When you raise your arms in the beginning movement, use that resting control of the muscle that gives the gentle fall of the t'ai chi arm, rolling your shoulders and bringing your head back to center. Remember to do it sequentially: shoulders, elbows, wrists, and finally fingertips. Then check how your head is resting into your floating spine.

Also be aware of the breathing that corresponds

to this rise and fall of your arms. The lift and the rise is the obvious place for the air to come in, and somewhere as you begin to come down, the exhalation begins. Many times I'm asked about the breathing pattern. "Are you breathing in or breathing out?" I have to say, "I don't know, I never stop to think." You don't stop at the height of your so-called stretch and decide; you must melt it together so that it becomes one flow. Before you know it you are coming down, and breathing out. Then somewhere you begin to rise and your lungs begin to expand. As you sink, the air comes out again. It will all happen together if you become really aware of your body as you move, without interfering with it.

After the beginning arm lift and fall, you move into the movement called Grasping the Sparrow's Tail. As your hands settle, find something in your body orientation that makes you want to yield to one side rather than the other side. Find something right now that you can identify without thinking "right." If you think "right" there will be a pause and a break in your movement flow. There must be something—maybe the sight of the person next to you, maybe the sound coming from the road, maybe the trees moving. Find something right now to make you feel an attraction to the right side, and go with that flow.

I have mentioned that in the form we always begin to the right side after the beginning arm lift. We don't know why—maybe one particular early ta'i chi master was left-handed so it goes right. Often I begin to the left and do the whole form left-sided. Sometimes I even begin the form at the end and do it backwards to the beginning. Some people will tell you that if you do this, your ch'i, your breath energy, will circulate "backwards" and mess you up. If you are keeping up a circular flow of energy, how can there be a "forwards" or "backwards"? If you are at one point in a circle you can go either way and arrive at the same point. Breathing out comes before *and* after breathing in. The only way you could do it "backwards" would be to breathe in when your lungs are already full and you need to breathe out, or to breathe out when the movement is expanding your chest.

Tomorrow morning when you come out and practice with me, begin by finding your center and your t'ai chi base. Then focus on your breathing and let it flow into the beginning arm lift and the movements that follow that, which are variations of the t'ai chi sphere.

Already you have quite a few specific things to work with in your morning practice. If you really follow the principles you have learned, and if I don't compare you with the form, I would say, "Oh, that looks very nice." If you get stuck, the t'ai chi sphere is always a good transition to bring you back into a nice looping feeling. Just move around and play with these motifs we have practiced and make your own transitions. Don't worry about what comes next. Why not put any two movements together if it feels right? If it doesn't feel right you can work out something in between, so that each one moves smoothly into the next.

I would like to see you moving on your own more every morning instead of just watching me. If we are all practicing together and aware of each other, we will trigger each other. If there is a rock here, a tree here, and a person here—somehow the rock has its rockness, the tree has its treeness, and you have your you-ness. That's what a t'ai chi practice looks like when you practice together. Everything should move on its own, and then they are working in harmony.

Right now, let your arm be arm. Let your neck be neck. And if neck and arm happen to move together, they make beautiful music. Your arms can become one curving line through your back. Your legs can connect through your pelvis like an arc. Let a curve in your body continue into another curve outside your body, perhaps into another body near you. All kinds of connections will happen easily if you let them—if your body is free of your dictating mind.

Everything that is happening in your body comes from one source: That same settling feeling that we

call t'ai, the middle-centered feeling in your physical/
mental self. If you are constantly in touch with that
source as you move, then the outside forces around
your moving body, all that is happening around you
will become a part of your sphere of movement.

When you observe nature and look at rocks and
waves, you realize that each has its own nature. The
wave is being wave and the rock is being rock. When
the wave and the rock come together they create
rock/wave, wave/rock. They have a separateness and
also a togetherness in which each one is very much
itself. If the wind comes blowing and the tree is there,
rooted down, then it becomes wind/tree, tree/
branch/wind. Human beings can move like all these
things. We can be rooted down like rock or tree, or
we can move like wind, like water.

III

We were talking last night about the origin of t'ai chi and the relationship between t'ai chi, tao, and the Chinese historical, political, and social situation. The t'ai chi concept goes way back to the beginnings of Chinese history, to an unrecorded time called the period of mythical rulers. One of them, Fu Hsi, created the t'ai chi symbol and the idea of the eight trigrams which have developed into the *I Ching*, the Book of Changes. T'ai goes back to the first moment a man feels a sense of himself and a need to orient himself in his environment.

Philosophy comes out of this search, this sense of questioning what life is all about. Out of this need, man creates different theories and concepts to make sense out of his world. The Chinese t'ai chi thought is not much different from some of the thoughts of the Greeks and Romans. For instance, there is the idea of Heraclitus that you never step into the same river twice, because the river flows and changes. This idea is the same as t'ai chi.

T'ai chi is also the basis of taoism, which parallels and complements confucianism. Confucianism has a way of structuring everything. It keeps human beings in harmony by establishing particular relationships between the king and his subject, father and son, older brother and younger, husband and wife—everything has its own place. It's a very nice idea until it becomes so rigid and tight that nobody can budge. It also becomes very superficial. Everybody is *supposed* to be loyal to his king and to be filial to his parents, and the wife must do everything for the husband—she never complains and always walks three paces behind. These restrictions structured everything so tightly that people were *screaming*—especially the people who were really creatively in tune with the natural flow of things.

To balance this extreme we had the development of taoism, which is exemplified by the teachings of Lao Tzu. Lao Tzu is probably a fictional name, because Lao Tzu means "old man." One theory is that his name was Lee and he was a very learned man, the curator for one of the archives. Another legend says that Lao Tzu was carried in the womb by his mother for eighty-one years, so he was born wise already. There are many stories, but they all agree that he was a very wise man who really understood nature. He and his students worked on clarifying and using the concept of tao.

The *Tao te Ching* is supposed to have been written either by him or by his students, or both. It has been developed throughout the years, and it has become one of the canons of scripture in Chinese philosophy. If we study the *Tao te Ching*, everything in it says t'ai chi. The text is a series of very short poems talking about paradox, the unknown, nature. It is so paradoxical and so difficult to translate that everybody has a new interpretation.

Later in the week I will spend a session doing calligraphy with you. I will illustrate within the calligraphy the intrinsicness and the essence of the Chinese language which is non-linear. The English language is linear. You may look at the word "love" and identify a certain feeling with the lines. But the essence—the l shape and o shape and the v shape and the e shape—is something completely abstract.

Although the Chinese culture is very old and some of it is very sophisticated and complex, the basic essence of the written language is still very primitive and concrete. Most characters developed out of sketches or line drawings of what they represent. So if you look into the strokes of the character itself you can often see deeper meanings in them. I will do some of this in the calligraphy session, and later I will translate some of the *Tao te Ching* for you.

The *Tao te Ching* always leaves room for interpretation and never finishes for you. It used to be traditional that you should always interpret it in your own words. Each time I translate it, I have to start all over again, within my understanding at the moment. It talks about being and non-being, action and nonaction—all these paradoxes of opposites. If you ask what is the literature of t'ai chi, it's the *Tao te Ching* and *I Ching*, the Book of Changes. Those are the two main scriptures in Chinese literature that are directly connected to the t'ai chi we are working on. In the *I Ching*, however, many interpretations and commentaries have been added by various scholars throughout the years, including Confucius and his many disciples. These additions often clutter the original taoist simplicity.

At that time, the taoists must have been like the original bohemians or hippies who just take off to do their thing. For instance, the Zen Buddhist called Han San, "the cold mountain," is a village idiot who laughs at the wind and smiles at the tiniest little thing. The taoists were simple people who could really identify with the simple life, and not let thinking trouble the process of living. They were the living/doing people, the people who allowed things to happen.

There are many basic concepts in tao that emerge in t'ai chi when you practice. One is the word pŭ, which means the original material, before it's trimmed and modified, fixed and polished. Sometimes we translate this as "uncarved block." It's the raw material before it is carved into an artistic form, the essence that exists before you change it. Learn the grain of the wood before you begin to carve it. Pŭ is the basic substance of the real you, before it's manicured or painted over. Expose your own basic essence before you clutter it up. Don't let all the external things blind you so that you lose the uncarved block within. This is what we are doing in t'ai chi. Every time we begin, we must find that uncarved original wood, that basic sense of what the human body is, that sense of being all together. We usually keep telling ourselves what we are, instead of just letting the pŭ emerge.

The Japanese concept wabi is similar. It is sometimes translated as "poverty," being content with the simple things so there is no extra stuff. If you look at t'ai chi as a movement form, you know how simple it is. It is one of the purest, most crystallized forms of movement. It's condensed into the most essential, basic elements of expression. It's all there.

Another idea is that we must return to being an infant again. Can you still breathe as freely as a baby? That's the child*like*ness we should maintain. We shouldn't be child*ish*. Child*like*ness is what we all enjoy. We want to keep that. We want to keep alive, with all the openness and sense of wonder about life and about ourselves. But we lose that as we grow up. We are afraid to appear awkward or ignorant—we want to be perfectly under control and pretend that we know everything.

Recently I went to a very incongruous event. A group of upper-middle-class white people sponsored a community concert called the American Black Theater of Jazz. They collected a group of entertainers from the old Apollo theater in Harlem. All these old performers were in their sixties and seventies. They were marvelous. The show opened with them parading around, wearing bright clothes, and it was fascinating. I applauded, I jumped up and down, I danced. Children were sitting there, and when I laughed, they looked at me and seemed to say, "When he laughs, maybe I can laugh." They were all such little stuffed-shirts, and I thought, "Oh, what have we done to our younger generation!" When I sit in a theater I find myself responding with a great deal of movement. People sitting next to me often resent my exuberance and seem to be saying, "What are you doing? You're disturbing me. Appreciate esthetic values!" Esthetics does not apply to you if you cannot move. When I dance, I want people to move with me. I am dancing *with* you; I don't dance to you or for you; it's not a matter of separation.

Recently a t'ai chi fad seems to be mushrooming in all the big cities. Everybody is taking t'ai chi and getting degrees in it—even junior and senior certificates. I'm glad that so many people are interested in this beautiful practice, but I'm a little worried about the bastardization of t'ai chi.

It's like the interest in judo and karate after the war. Because the big, tall American soldiers got thrown all over by a tiny little Japanese judo expert, suddenly everyone became interested in judo. First there was judo training in the army and then it mushroomed all over. In every big city there are judo studios everywhere. Every YMCA has a karate club, and every school has one. But often most of the appeal of this training is just the showing-off of strength. When I first came to this country, I went to a few studios, just to find out what they were like. Most of the students never had the vaguest idea of what the *essence* of judo was all about. All they knew was how to throw somebody over. They wore their Japanese practice clothes, and they strutted and grunted. This kind of development went on and on and then pretty soon, of course, the thoughtful people would say, "Oh, that's terrible, it can't be like this."

And now t'ai chi emerges, it slowly sneaks out. T'ai chi has always been in the background. The older men in Chinatowns have always practiced t'ai chi, but they were never conspicuous; they practiced very quietly where nobody noticed. There's so much confusion about t'ai chi, sometimes I begin to wonder if I should use the words t'ai chi at all. It sounds so foreign, so exotic, you tend to think you're getting something very different, very special. T'ai chi is not something that differs from what you already have. I always say I do not teach. There's no way to teach. What is teaching? I don't say, "I'm a t'ai chi master because I learned it when I was a child, so I have it and you don't have it, and I'm going to teach it to you and show you how difficult it is." If I did that you would get very frustrated and say, "What if I cannot hang onto it? Tell me what I am doing wrong." A t'ai chi master would tell you that you're doing nothing wrong but you just don't have it yet.

It takes years and years to fully discover t'ai chi. You cannot just learn life instantly. Life is to be lived. You might think "If I find a good teacher, if I read a good book, I will eventually become very wise, and I will have conquered all the difficulties in life." If you do that, then what's next? Boredom. The physical understanding of movement that we call t'ai chi can help you to understand and face the difficulties in your life, but it won't eliminate all your problems.

The concept of t'ai chi only means a way of learning how to regain balance again. It is a way to come back to yourself from all the conflicts and confusions that we feel every day in our lives. T'ai chi does not mean oriental wisdom or something exotic. It is the wisdom of your own senses, your own body and mind together as one process.

Many people think t'ai chi just means that phrase of movement called the t'ai chi ch'uan. People find that by practicing it they can cure a lot of psychosomatic diseases. They begin to feel they can breathe better and sleep better. When they look at a master they are amazed and happy to hear that this master is actually 90 but he looks only 60. That doesn't mean anything. That's only a fringe benefit. If that master is very good with t'ai chi and he looks young, that has nothing to do with *you*.

The essence of t'ai chi is really to help you to get acquainted with your *own* sense of potential growth, the creative process of just being you. T'ai chi helps you to be you and to let that sense of wonder and development and constant joy of changing happen in you. T'ai chi is a discipline that you as a person, as a human being, can begin to dig into and practice, and it will serve you.

Several days ago a man came to me after watching us practicing for about an hour and said, "I enjoy watching very much. Whatever you're doing reminds me of wild animals. You have the same kind of freedom and balance and rhythm. But the spine of the trained racehound is different." I said, "Yes. Racehounds are trained to achieve a particular purpose, to run fast. Hopefully, we will not become racehounds." In t'ai chi, we do not train ourselves so our bodies are distorted in one way to achieve something special. Then the body looks like something trained and limited, a result of working so hard to achieve something special, to become an image that you *think* you want to be.

In the beginning I was in danger of being trained like a hound because I wanted to be the best of that particular school of t'ai chi ch'uan. Each one of us probably has that need and has the desire to get the *best* master, the *best* teacher. But you don't really learn from your master; you learn from your own body as you practice. I never teach the form exactly the way it was handed down to me, because after I have practiced so many years I don't really remember exactly how the master asked me to do that first gesture. If you really learn t'ai chi well, it becomes your own creation.

The first t'ai chi master created t'ai chi out of the enlightenment of his own nature, out of his awareness of his body. He learned from the wisdom of his own body and his identification with nature, and then he developed this beautiful movement phrase. I would say it's pure movement because it's not cluttered with outside knowledge, or with hopes or other people's expectations. T'ai chi at its best, in its purest form, is almost invisible—so little to look at, so small you do not admire it for its fanciness. And it's so elusive you cannot hang on to it—it does not have a set, dead structure. You just don't know where you are. The only way you can find where you are is to dive right into the middle of it, and learn from *you* doing it. You can't learn much from beautiful ideas alone. All that knowledge comes from outside and does not really serve you.

I want you to dig into the movement of t'ai chi not as a foreign product but as something very familiar to you as human bodies. We all have two arms, two legs and a spine. Our ranges may be different, but basically the connection is the same and the unity is the same. The difficulty is that we are not as free, as open, as natural as we used to be when we were first born. We're not breathing like an infant any more, we are not moving naturally like wild animals, the way the man/animal should. We are domesticated. We are already stuck with too many straight-jackets we have to wear—too many bows and pins and folds on our body. So this is an unlearning process; it's not a learning-*more* process. If you are here to learn more, then you must curve around to feel you are learning less.

This has everything and nothing to do with what we call t'ai chi ch'uan which as a form becomes an achievement. You can learn a movement phrase because your body and mind are acquainted with that flow, and you can repeat and duplicate that particular pattern. But that's different from t'ai chi. I use the form to demonstrate, to illustrate the flow of t'ai chi visually and physically, but our goal is not to merely learn that beautiful phrase of movement. That phrase was created by a taoist who was a very enlightened man. But I want you to learn to do your own t'ai chi. If you really understand t'ai chi you will be able to create t'ai chi ch'uan instantaneously.

Do t'ai chi ch'uan your own way and it will eventually look like the t'ai chi ch'uan that original t'ai chi master developed and handed down to us. Even this particular form that we all come to know has many variations. Unfortunately, when each master begins to teach, he may use *his* master's teaching method as he remembers it, instead of sharing with you out of his own experience *now*. Another problem is that the master may try to teach you what he can do now as a result of years of practice, instead of showing you a process that can gradually lead you to this.

He may think that if you just keep working and working to fit into that form that someday you will find the freedom—like practicing piano scales. But think how many people practice scales, and how many Horowitzes or Rubinsteins do we have? Do you really believe that you can become a great artist simply by practice, practice, practice? I think not; I think there must also be a lot of inner growth and vitality along with discipline. An athlete may require a trainer to keep him on a schedule, keep him going. But without an inner sense of wanting to work, a trainer can beat you to death without getting you anywhere.

As we work, we use the form as a guide. It is something to work *with*, not something you learn to show off. The form is a process that serves you, not an adornment like a beautiful art work you buy and bring back to hang on your wall. That's like going to Japan and bringing back a scroll and feeling that you have brought a bit of the orient back with you. You can enjoy that but it's still not really yours; it's still outside you. I hope you don't carry home a phrase of movement so you can say, "I have gone to a workshop and now I know something called t'ai chi—see how special I am."

If you really learn t'ai chi, it comes out of the body so naturally it looks like you just made it up on the spot. You begin and finish not even knowing you have done it. If someone is watching you, they don't even see you have done it. It takes years of practice to reach this. There is no instant achievement. The true discipline is something that you *live with* and which becomes an ongoing thing, a way of life with you.

Most of the time we want *not* to change. We think we can find something nice and secure, and we want to hang onto it. We forget that the constant can only build upon change. The world keeps changing, so if you try to hang onto the moment, you're lost. But if you follow the changing moment, then you reach a constant moving. You go with what happens; you carry that sense of stability with your moving self. You experience both the movement and stillness together. If you apply this idea to your daily thinking and your way of perceiving your existence, then it can help you. T'ai chi is a philosophy that starts with the basic not-knowing, the basic relaxation of giving it. This can begin with just sitting here not trying too hard to listen to what I say and not trying to take mental notes. If you feel comfortable not knowing, you get to know the unknown much faster, without effort.

Most of us are always rushing. We try so hard to find *the* answer, and we seldom have the patience to wait for it. You are never going to get anywhere anyway. Can you accept that? Can you really accept that? The moment you do, BOOM! Life opens up. It's very ironic because if you're really in a rush to know what life is all about, then just *do* it and get it over with. You could be born, take the first breath, give one loud cry—AHHHHHH—and die. That's very efficient. That was really a success, wasn't it?

In the aikido session last Friday they were doing touching and sensing with their hands. They were trying to feel energy coming out of their palms. Sometimes you do, sometimes you don't, and sometimes you *think* you do, but anyway it's a nice image to help you feel the energy of the pushing hand. If you do this as you push, then it won't become just a rigid, dead gesture. As you practice, every once in a while you may get a little tingling sensation as if you feel something coming out of your palms. When you push, don't let the energy stop. It never stops. It either flows up or down or sideways, and always comes back in a curve.

If you do this pushing with a feeling of sending energy out, then it is alive. It may help if you grunt a little as you push. Grunting is almost like forcing, but if you let that force flow out, then that's where the ch'i, the breath energy, is. Don't get congested, don't get constipated. Grunt from deep in your belly. Give birth to the grunt and feel the energy right here in your center.

Now stand near a wall, and push against it. How

are you using your energy? The deeper you settle into your base, the better. Find that position in which you can push with maximum energy, from the tant'ien. Now, when you feel the complete resistance of that wall, instead of wasting that energy, pull your hands back and bring it back into you. Don't lose it. If you had the strength of Samson, that wall would fall down. When that happens, don't fall forward; conserve and retain that energy by bringing it back down into your center. Be sure to keep your back straight, so the recoil energy flows directly back through your spine to the tant'ien where the ch'i reservoir is. When you recoil, the elbow comes back in and sinks—can you feel that? Don't push so much that you tighten and can't recoil.

Now pair up with someone else and push strongly against his hands in the same way. Now when one of you suddenly pulls his hands back, the other should be able to pull back with that same recoiling energy. If you fall forward, then you're not staying centered as you push.

Now separate and do this pushing and recoil alone. Just push the space in front of you away, and let the energy recoil back to you. This will be very helpful for those of you who are having problems with the beginning sequential resting arm movement.

This is also a technique to not waste your energy. Even when you do a sharp kick in karate, after that kick there is that recoiling. Do a small kick, as if you are shaking off a loose shoe. Notice that the recoil, the bouncing back, is something that happens by itself. You don't have to *do* it, you just *allow* it. After the rebound your leg is bent a little, ready for another kick. If you just kick out, then you have spent your energy uselessly. But if you send it out and then bring it back, then you use it but you don't lose it.

One principle in the practice of t'ai chi is understanding what you can do with your energy without wasting it into action. Then you have this constant sense of possibilities, and if the need comes you can respond to it instantly, without thinking. One of my friends studied judo for years and years. She was waiting for the chance to use it, but for a long time nobody tried to attack her. Then one day somebody grabbed her in a parking lot—and she slugged him with her purse! And then she thought, "Oh! What happened to my judo?" She must have been practicing judo as if it were an isolated thing. We should always practice to let the immediacy of the moment come through. Then you always have a sense of what you are doing *now*. When you go through your t'ai chi in the morning, it's not a matter of just following through that established pattern you have learned, but of each time letting the next movement happen for you. If you get stuck somewhere, don't follow the mind saying "It should go that way," but just follow that moment, *now*. If you do the movement correctly, it will take you there. That's the beauty of t'ai chi: it's a natural flow.

This kind of happening that is so spontaneous is called Tse-jan in Chinese, "self-so-ness"—or sono-mama in Japanese. When the leaves fall from the trees, they follow the wind, and if they happen to drop on the water they just follow the currents. A leaf does not fight and say, "I want to go back on the branch," or "There's a dirty spot; I don't want to land there." Your movement and your life can also become an easy happening that follows the wind and the currents.

There are many natural metaphors in t'ai chi, and a number of motifs are named after animals. One is called White Crane Cools Its Wings. When we do this movement we are not trying to imitate the outer shape of the crane, but rather to get a feeling of what flying must be like. If you are a bird, you have a very concentrated center of gravity and your wing motion playing with space becomes very important.

Now extend your arms to the sides and play with pushing down the space with your arms as you rise. Feel the bounce and resilience in your legs as you move up with each downward arm motion, and settle down as your arms rise. Now experiment with pushing down very close alongside your body. As you feel your body coming up it's like squeezing through a very tight space. You cannot lift yourself by your own bootstraps, but if you push down against something else, then you can lift yourself easily. The more you relate your movement to something outside, the more release you feel. As you go up, sink down; as you go down, lift up. It sounds contradictory, but if you didn't have the down to push against, you couldn't possibly go up. You have to sense the connection, the yin/yang relatedness of these apparent opposites.

There is a story of one famous t'ai chi master who had acquired a high degree of instantaneous resilience in his body. A small bird resting in his palm was unable to take off because of the complete lack of resistance in the hand. The bird could not muster enough rebound from the palm to spring off. At the same time, the t'ai chi master learned and identified with the bird in its preparation for flight. He sank toward the ground as the bird pushed into his palm, and he experienced in his body the sensation of the bird ready to take flight.

Now move your arms in circles and see if you are making the connection between your ups and downs. Feel this circular movement in your body also. This circle may become very small and concentrated, but it should always be there.

Now try swimming motions with your arms and feel the water you are pushing away as you swim forward. Twist into the movement with your body and feel how your pushing the water advances you. Now do a backstroke, and be sure to rotate your arms so that the palm faces down as you pull the water towards you. See if you can rotate your arms without turning the body too much.

If you walk forward now as you continue the backstroke arm-circles, this becomes the movement called White Crane Cools His Wings. Your arms are stirring the space around you. Keep all your joints relaxed, and let the two arms connect in one sweeping motion. The arm moving back is ready to receive whatever energy comes from behind you as you move forward. The other arm takes care of whatever comes from in front, so both back and front are protected. Get this all-around feeling of the sphere of protected space around you. Feel your legs testing the ground beneath you as you walk, and feel the space in front and above and behind with your arms. The arm movements will naturally open your body to the side and back as you walk. If you really get this feeling of all-around readiness, then your movement will be vital; you won't just wave your arms like spinning wheels. This forward movement then circles back into the next motif which is essentially the motion of drawing a bow and letting the arrow shoot forward as you step backward.

It's difficult to keep the movement going in your whole body at once, particularly when you're first learning. If you focus too much attention on the movement of one hand, then the movement tends to stop elsewhere, and the other hand may become like a dead branch. I can usually tell when you start to think, because these dead spots show up somewhere in your body. Then you become separated and fragmented, and you lose the feeling of oneness, of moving together all over.

One of the best ways to become connected in the body is through t'ui sho which means "pushing hands." Pair up with someone else and stand facing him with your right foot forward. Gently touch your right wrists together and begin to move your hands in a small horizontal counter-clockwise circle. In this basic, first experience of t'ui sho you use your arm as an extension of half a circle and use this revolving hand to connect your body energy with your partner's.

There is nothing like working with another person to point out how you are resistant, and where your thinking and doing are in conflict. I used this one time in a couples workshop, and I practice this with my wife when we feel crossed and in conflict. She's a very headstrong woman and sometimes when we disagree I say, "Suzanne, let's do t'ui sho." She says,

"I don't want to do t'ui sho; I've had enough of your encounter things." And I say, "I don't blame you. But we got to do t'ui sho because I can't talk to you now." So we do t'ui sho. And as we do t'ui sho we go through some of the arguments in our minds. And before you know it, certain things seem to come this way and certain ideas seem to go that way. Certain ideas sort of loop around and get stuck in a little whirlpool and others come back. We take quite a while to do this. It's a way of arranging things and transforming that mind process into a movement process.

If I'm resisting too much while doing t'ui sho, then I find myself tensing up—making a special point to relax or trying to show that I'm really completely free and open about some particular idea. As I'm stressing a point that I don't really believe, I find myself pushing harder and harder. So it's very revealing. The movement says *so* clearly what's wrong with an encounter, without having to say it in words. If you work with somebody who is very, very rigid, he may say, "Well, why don't you follow me? You're resisting." If he feels you resisting, then you're being just as rigid as he is. Don't fight him. Give in to him, and gradually this imbalance will be resolved. Nobody is yin or yang. Nobody is completely dominant or passive. You have to find that mutual point to begin.

Now separate for a moment and find your own center by pressing your palms hard against each other with the fingertips up, like an isometric exercise. Now let your elbows sink, and let your hands rise slowly up the center line, ascending like a praying gesture. Do this several times.

Now do a similar upward push with your partner. Face each other again with your right feet forward and push your right hands together. Now let your elbows slowly sink and feel your hands rise up the mutual center-line between you. As your hands rise higher, let them separate and curve out to your right and down. Continue this curve until your fingertips meet again, and your hands rise up the center-line between you.

Now let's return to the t'ui sho. If we both push our right hands against each other rigidly, it's like the old-fashioned contest to see who is physically stronger. We get to a standstill. If we can mutually reduce that energy very slowly, we will get to a point where we are pushing very lightly against each other. Now the slightest extra energy from either side will begin the circular t'ui sho movement.

I want all of you to try this. Find a mutual center and push against each other strongly until your energy becomes equal. And then, very slowly, very peacefully, reduce your energy until you are touching lightly against each other. Do this slowly, and let whatever happens take over. Whoever happens to be outgoing yang at the moment will begin to move out a little, and then curve back into the yielding yin. As this happens, you have already begun that t'ui sho circle.

This circular soft flow of t'ui sho is not easy. It is usually considered "advanced work" that the master teaches only after you have learned the whole form and you are considered quite good in the technique. The master works with you to reflect your tension and difficulties, and gets his energy into you to help balance you. In the old way of teaching t'ai chi nothing is ever explained, so it would be harmful for two beginners to do t'ui sho together. Beginners tend to discuss and analyze too much; they would just confuse themselves. However, I use t'ui sho to immediately show how the other person's body reflects your own tension. When you do partner-work, you are doing yin/yang movement right away. The yin energy and the yang energy must work together, and the real t'ai chi happens.

T'ui sho can get very complex, very involved. Starting with this simple circular pattern, it can develop into an S-shape, a figure-eight, using both hands, arms, elbows, shoulders, hips—eventually the whole body is involved all over. The whole idea is the image of the amoeba. If you push it this way, it just bounces out that way. The body must work that fluidly. Especially if you think of the body as so many joints and awkward places, then it is very beautiful to watch.

When you do t'ui sho really well, you arrive at a point where the form completely disappears. Eventually you may move into a form we call san sho which means "a free dispersing hand." It's a very free, clean form—the kind of open improvisation that happens when everything is clear, settled, and centered. Then whatever you do reflects this enlightened state of t'ai chi.

There is also a set, definitely structured t'ui sho form that is called san sho. You don't have to get stuck with the form because it is only a point of departure for what you do. When you see the old masters practice, they first do the form and then they begin to just let go and improvise. It's very beautiful to watch, because it's as if some new creation continually unfolds in front of you.

I experienced san sho when I was in Taiwan three years ago. I managed to be allowed into one of the oldest t'ai chi societies. As these old masters went about their t'ui sho, I was surprised by their casual conversation: "How's wife? How's family? How's business?" Their movement became very complex and involved. When I was finally invited to join in, I was too anxious to show my best. I tried too hard to become a part of their movement, and I couldn't make contact. I was trying too hard to think what I should be doing and panicked. They enjoyed it tremendously when I got lost. Finally, I gave up trying and went with the flow, and the flow caught up with me! I will never forget the gentle smiles on those old faces as they saw me succeed.

The taoist, Lieh-tzu, describes this feeling beautifully. After ten years of practicing meditation and moving, he comes home feeling as if he is an old dried leaf separating from the tree, just fluttering to and fro with the wind. He is floating about, and he doesn't know if the wind is riding him or he is riding the wind.

"It was then that the eye was like the ear, and the ear like the nose, and the nose like the mouth; for they were all one and the same. The mind was in rapture, the form dissolved, and the bones and flesh all thawed away; and I did not know how the frame supported itself and what the feet were treading upon. I gave myself away to the wind, eastward or westward, like leaves of a tree."

IV

During the first few days of your practice you are usually reluctant and self-conscious, and you try to program yourself. The letting-go process is not happening as much as it should be. This morning Arlene said that when we were doing the beginning breathing it was so cold outside that she had to keep moving around. She didn't have time to worry about whether she was doing it right or wrong and it came easier to her. This is exactly what t'ai chi should be.

I often encounter people who have done some t'ai chi, and carry it around with them like a burden. When you look at them moving, it's obvious that there is a kind of sad self-consciousness and awkwardness. If you feel awkward doing t'ai chi, you're doing it wrong. The minute you feel awkward, don't insist upon achieving the form—come back to your naturalness before you continue.

T'ai chi is the purest, most natural organic form. The human body should adapt to it very quickly and easily—if we don't interfere with the body's natural flow. But the society we live in confines us in many ways; we lose our spontaneity and natural freedom of movement. We are all cramped, braced, with constraints on our body and mind. This is why we are all interested in unwinding. Someone said, "This unwinding process is very tiring." And I said, "Are you *trying* to learn?" And she said, "Well, maybe I am." Don't try; then it won't be tiring. This is why I'm only giving you a little bit new each day.

We all look at children and say, "Ah, how beautifully they move." But then some well-meaning parents send their child to the ballet school too early. She puts on toe shoes and a little tutu, and pretty soon the child doesn't have a single spontaneous movement, because of feeling so self-conscious, always looking in the mirror. All our lives we have been told not to express ourselves openly, so we keep putting a clamp here, a brace there, a staple there, and soon our bodies are full of all these mental and physical congestions. By the time we are adults we feel so stiff that our bodies can't give. We trip over things, we get hurt, we become shells, always fighting against the outside form. We manipulate ourselves in order to fit a mold, and then our body fights back against this unnatural distortion.

What you need is an acceptance of yourself as you are. You are like a seed. You don't know what you're going to be when spring comes—maybe a chrysanthemum, or an orchid, or maybe just a plain dandelion. Do you want to know the outcome of the flowering that much? What about simply letting yourself be during the flowering process? *Be* with the process and *enjoy* it. When the flower comes to full bloom, it is usually the last part of your life, and you're ready to go to seed. You've spent all your life looking, working, worrying, fighting for that last moment of flowering which is going to be a glorious display. Because of intellectual ideas we are always aiming towards some gorgeous flower that each one of us has in mind. Most of the time we don't become that exact flower, and we are very unhappy. Life is the process, the preparing for the flowering. If seeds had goals, there wouldn't be very many flowers.

Two years ago, I met a Tibetan man, Sonam Kazi. He was the interpreter for the Dalai Lama at one time, but he wears American suits and looks like a businessman. He has bright twinkling eyes and is very quiet. I invited him and his family to the San Diego zoo. It was a very busy day so we had to wait in this little labyrinth for forty minutes to get on the tour bus to take us around. Everybody else was irritated and impatient. He was smiling at me and said, "Well, this is like the bardo." He was speaking about the *Tibetan Book of the Dead*, the intermediate stages, the forty-nine days between death and re-birth. The Tibetan concept, of course, is that nothing ends and everything is cyclical.

He talked about knowledge. "Don't try to learn knowledge as if you are driving with your defrosters off in the snow. Because this knowledge will keep sticking on your windshield. Pretty soon you can't see anything, and you will become blind and confused. This kind of knowledge never becomes a part of you: it's between you and the world." Unfortunately we usually seek knowledge from outside of us instead of inside.

He made another parallel when he saw me holding my arms in front of my body in a circle. "Now this looks like the opening of a pot of boiling hot water, with steam and energy moving up. True knowledge is like snowflakes falling into the pot. They melt and disappear as they hit the surface of the water." You don't see what you really learn—it dissolves in you and becomes you and changes you.

You don't have to say, "I have read this book, that book." That is all on the bookshelf. That is all in a computer somewhere. That kind of knowledge has nothing to do with you; it is a burden. If you learn to absorb knowledge and make it your own, then it only emerges when you need it. We talk about drawing upon experiences to face problems. In one sense, whatever you have experienced before must be a part of you. You don't have to constantly recognize it and talk about it. Real knowledge is invisible. If you absorb experience and let it dissolve in you, then you're uncluttered and you have an emptiness that is receptive to the situation now.

If you come with a full cup, there's no room for me to pour in any more tea. Most of us have this problem. Perhaps I have tasted jasmine tea; I like it, so I go around with a full cup of jasmine. If I drink the

jasmine and digest it, instead of carrying it around
saying "Yes, I understand jasmine," then I have room
for something new and fresh. If I have an empty cup,
maybe someone would offer me some oolong or
darjeeling!

This is what I am hoping to do in my t'ai chi and
dancing. Every day I get up and begin dancing all
over again from scratch. It would be an illusion to
think that because yesterday I practiced and I was
able to turn in the air three times, so today I can get
up and do it again. I'm just sitting here. How do you
know I can do three turns in mid-air? You can only
know when it happens. What you can do with your
body is invisible. Each time I have to go back to the
completely empty floor and start again. Then that *now*
movement happens. I am able to spin and turn and
enjoy the feeling of the dance.

Energy and movement should be like that. You
shouldn't have a stuck-on phrase or style to show you
know t'ai chi, or have to quote many t'ai chi masters
or particular passages of t'ai chi concepts. We can all
do that. When we work, we need to dig into the movement and really do it, and then let it enter us so we
will have our own kind of satori. "Ah! Yes! I understand this." You don't even have to translate this experience or talk about it—"Oh, this is just like that."
We do this all the time; we compare notes. It's fine as
long as the experience doesn't get lost in the words.
It's even better if we compare notes through movement, without words. In t'ui sho, for instance, we
share what we feel and perceive in the body.

Living is a continuous rebirth process. If you
learn something today, tomorrow morning you have to
start all over again. If you accept that, then there's no
need for a binding structure. A good structure should
have the flexibility to change and adapt. It will emerge
when you practice, but it will look and feel different
every day.

Yesterday I asked why can't we do the whole t'ai
chi ch'uan in the reverse of the way it is handed
down? Why does the first movement always have to

turn to the right? Barry was telling us the story about the woman who always cut off the end of the ham and somebody asked why she did it. She said, "Well, I don't know, my mother always did it that way." And they asked her mother and she said, "I don't know, *my* mother always did it." And they asked grandma, and she said, "Well, I did it because otherwise it wouldn't fit in my biggest pot."

I was born in Shanghai during the war. The Japanese were bombing the city and everybody was gone. My mother was in the hospital, but all the nurses and doctors were gone, so my grandmother delivered me. Right after that we got on a boat to go to Hong Kong and the boat sank. All of us were in the water for four days. Finally we were rescued and taken to a refugee camp. After a few days we went to southern China and after that from one village to another, all over. It was lucky for me and my brothers and sisters because we were able to really live with nature like the Chinese peasants. As I grew up, I was able to absorb quite a bit of the earth and the ways of the simple people into my own sensing and feeling. One of the things that ties us together as people is the simplicity and closeness to nature, because we can all sense and feel that unity. If I had lived in Shanghai I would probably have become very westernized. When I went to high school in Taiwan I did become very westernized. I listened to all the American top tunes, I wore blue jeans and colorful shirts and I rode a motorcycle. Anything western was fun and glamorous. I went to all the American movies and then, of course, I had to come to America.

When I came to this country I was sixteen and couldn't speak English very well. I plunged into American college, anxious to learn and become as American as possible, wanting so much to fit into this country. I forgot all about what I knew in the East, and just wanted to achieve, achieve, achieve. I got my degrees; I made it to the best of concert halls, and I got salutory reviews. I became a performer with a lot of grinding, pushing and body-hurting, trying to match that standard of what I thought a concert artist-dancer was supposed to be. I practiced ten hours a day and just worked and worked until my body felt exhausted. My body hurt and I had knee problems, hip problems, and ankle problems, like most dancers in this country. I kept saying to myself that if I work this hard, I must be getting better. I bit my tongue and said, "This is part of the game, you know. We have to suffer. We artists . . . nobody understands how we suffer." It's a very sad way of saying that you have to get somewhere.

I think most of us feel we have to work so hard to get somewhere—somewhere that you think you want to be, or somebody has told you long ago that you should be. Then you get there and you realize it's really not what you want; the bottom drops out and you don't know what you're doing. I realized that I wasn't getting any return from all that grabbing, reaching and striving. I didn't feel any energy coming back to me.

The only thing that kept me going at that time was the creative part of my work in dance. I began to create dances and I found that the only things that really made sense—what I wanted to dance and I felt honest doing—were usually things related to my childhood in China. My Oriental background was emerging and being expressed through my western way of exploration and expression in dancing. In a sense I was beginning to do ta'i chi again without even realizing the connection. I hadn't done t'ai chi at all in the years I was here.

I was invited to perform as a debut soloist at Jacob's Pillow Dance Festival in Massachusetts. It's very famous and important; if you dance there you have "emerged." Ted Shawn, the director of the place, automatically put down on the marquee, "Al Huang—Chinese dancer." I was very offended. I said, "Well, what do you mean I'm Chinese dancer? I'm not doing ethnic dance! I am not doing fluttering dance. Just because I'm Chinese I'm not doing Chinese dance. I don't want people to anticipate me doing lantern dance and scarf dance and all those things. I'm doing me, me, me!" I was very anxious to be me. And after a while I realized, "Well, what's the difference? What's the problem? Am I resisting the Chinese part of me because maybe I am still not identifying myself or settling in this foreign land? Maybe that's it."

So at the height of my Westernization my path began to curve back toward the East. I was trying to recapture what I had learned as a child in the villages in China. So I said to myself, "Well, why do I resist? I really have to get back to my heritage." I did one dance called Cicada Song, based on the life cycle of the seventeen-year locust, which is a typical poetic Chinese metaphor. I did a dance, Butterfly Dream, which is based on the paradoxical folk story about Chuang Tzu, a taoist. He repeatedly dreamed that he was flying, fluttering away as a butterfly and it bothered him so he went to Lao Tzu. Lao Tzu said, "Well, what are you worrying about? How do you know you're not a butterfly dreaming that you are a man? What makes you think you are dreaming butterfly? Maybe right now your human life is but a moment of a butterfly's dream?"

I began to realize that I was finding my own synthesis of East and West. All of us have to find our own way of coming back to our center. Some of us have a harder time than others. I was very fortunate because just at that time I received a grant from the Ford Foundation to do comparative study in the Arts. I went back to Taiwan for a year to teach at the College of Chinese Culture and the Foo Hsing opera school. I also had a chance to really recapture my t'ai chi by studying with the masters there, and I learned the sword practice, which is another outgrowth of t'ai chi.

That was the beginning of my return to the East. It happened to be a geographical one, too, but it didn't have to be. When I came back to the U.S. things began to really settle. That's when I started to give workshops for growth centers. I encountered Alan Watts, and what I was doing in movement followed what he was talking about in words. He is a man of language; he uses it most beautifully. In our joint workshops when the words get too thick, then we make the words come alive through movement. We dance together. Eventually we always get stuck talking, so we play to keep body and mind moving together.

Things began to happen in my dancing, too, as I worked to find a synthesis of East and West in me. T'ai chi became more and more important to me. It continues to help me find my balance and center. The more I practice t'ai chi, the more I absorb t'ai chi, the easier it becomes and the more dancing becomes a joy and a sharing. My concerts now start with t'ai chi dance. I dance sometimes in silence, sometimes to ocean music, birds, and water falling, whatever I find that feels right. I talk to the audience about t'ai chi and I invite them to dance with me and we share. And then after they get into it, I do more theatrical dancing. So t'ai chi works in my life as a dancer, performer, teacher.

T'ai chi is an opening-up process. It applies to all of us, all the time. If you are a potter, use it in your centering of the clay. If you are a painter, use it with your brush. There can be a lot of t'ai chi in science and engineering, too. The book called *The Tao of Science*—by an M.I.T. professor, R.G.H. Siu—shows how these ideas apply to science as well as arts and movement. Science has a way of understanding nature and trying to go one step beyond. All our most accomplished scientists get to the point where they reach the unknown again. Suddenly they become very open, very t'ai chi, very mystical. They do not say, "I have more brain, so I can conquer. I understand everything, so I can manipulate the universe."

In all this there is a way of receiving and giving that has no ending. When I first encountered situations like meeting people twice my age with much more experience in different professions, I hesitated, thinking "What do I have to share?" Now I know I don't have to assume that I have more to say or less to say than you, so I lose this hesitation. We are all on an equal basis. I learn as much from you as you learn from me.

This afternoon we have a free open period. I would like you to do a bit of exploring in your own way, to discover how your thoughts and your movements are interconnected. Whether you are swimming or walking, or driving on the road, concentrate on transferring your mind process into what you are *doing*. For instance, as you drive, many thoughts may stick in your mind. If you turn a curve, let some of these thoughts curve too. When you turn another curve, let other thoughts flow out that way. This can help simplify you, and it also relaxes you, so you don't get tense driving long distances. Because my wife doesn't drive, when we go across the country, I usually drive eight or more hours a day. When I move in this way I don't get tired.

Last Friday instead of taking the shortcut from San Francisco, I took the long, winding coast route. Instead of trying to rush and hang on to the wheel, I try to really feel the road. I'm moving the wheel and the wheel is moving me, and I'm doing my t'ai chi. Try going from your room to the lodge or to the baths with t'ai chi. Practice t'ai chi going downhill, on uneven terrain. Don't rely on the teacher or the master who often leads you by the nose. The sooner you can put t'ai chi movement into your own understanding of what you are doing, the better.

Try this process in whatever you are doing this afternoon, and explore what your movement can reveal to you, and perhaps resolve for you. Don't stop the flow. Don't stop to think, and don't hold back. When you move, don't stop and say, "What comes next?"—*do* it. Notice the correspondence between the movement part of your activity and your thinking and your ideas.

I very seldom work on personal problems with a participant because I usually don't find it's necessary. In t'ai chi we do not recognize problems. There is no problem. The minute you recognize it, it emerges, and then you may get stuck in it. I find that if I don't focus on a problem it has a way of settling by itself—without my disturbing it and pushing it by saying, "Why do you do that? How come you are resistant?" Then t'ai chi is not working for either of us.

I would like you to create a focus for yourself on the spot *as you do it.* If you set up goals ahead of time, they will blind you to what is happening at the moment, and the strain of trying to achieve your goal tends to make you tense and rigid and closed. Your focusing on goals separates you from true learning, which is simply your awareness of the day-to-day doing.

Let's say that you decide that your goal is to learn ta'i chi within five years, so you discipline yourself and practice like mad. You make yourself get up every morning to do it, and again before you go to sleep. Maybe you practice once more in the middle of the day. You are afraid if you go on a weekend trip that you will have no time and space for it and you will lose it. But if you lose it in three days' time you never really had it anyway, except superficially. If you always think of the outcome, then you can't be fully involved in what you are doing now. You are reaching and grabbing for the future which is beyond your grasp, and you miss what is within your reach in the present. Since you aren't getting anything, you reach harder and miss even more. You will find that nothing satisfies you, so you keep reaching out for a new guru, a new method, a new answer.

If you are lucky, you may discover for yourself that this reaching out for an answer and trying so hard is what separates you from your own experience and creates the problem. T'ai chi is a discipline that can help you settle into the experience of your body and your surroundings and re-establish contact with what is happening *now.* Then you can move out from this solid foundation of your ongoing experience.

When I learned t'ai chi as a child I had no goal. When I was five I didn't know I was going to come and teach at Esalen. I had no idea and I didn't care.

I just learned t'ai chi. And then in high school I became very un-t'ai chi, very Westernized, very separated. I became a goal-getter. I had to play the school game. I had to go to college. I had to pass the entrance examination to go abroad to study. Then I studied architecture, engineering, theater, and dance —always for degrees: bachelor's, master's, still trying to get hold of something. And then my life changed, and all the other disciplines didn't make any sense. The dancing discipline, the moving discipline was the only thing that really stayed with me.

Now t'ai chi is again the way it used to be with me when I was a child. If I can share this with you, fine. But mainly t'ai chi is for *me*. It is not just a tool to become a t'ai chi master so I can fly around the country and give workshops at nice places like Esalen. T'ai chi should be yours for you, too. It's not a matter of learning t'ai chi so that you can think you are slightly ahead of somebody else in the search for enlightenment. The discipline of t'ai chi can serve you right away, like this morning, and last night when you were having fun dancing and feeling alive, being a human body. You realize that the unlearning process is fun. It's not losing something: It's a *good* feeling to be empty again.

Last night, in between dancing, I went down to the baths and I sat there soaking. In the next tub, in the dark, there was a very heated discussion. There were voices coming out very strong, very absolute. One young man was saying, "I know something that you don't know—this country is owned by twenty families, for instance the DuPont family, blah blah blah." So he knows all the answers. At the same time a young man stepped into my pool, looked at me and said, slowly and softly, "Hi . . . You Buddhist?" I said, "Sometimes." And he said, "You do yoga?" I said, "Sometimes." He said, "I want to do yoga *all* my life. How do you do it?" I said, "Just do it." He said "Ohhhhh . . . Just do it. Oh, that's *beautiful*." So he's ignorant; he knows no answers. We were all floating there—with all the answers and no answers.

And what really happens, I think, is we know some of the answers sometimes, but most of the time we don't know the answers. It's a flow, it's not the yin *or* the yang. Sometimes we are attracted to an outgoing yang feeling. At other times we get to the point where we want some real sense of feeling of ourselves, so we turn inward in a yin way. When that becomes empty we reach out again. So you keep moving, and it's this interchanging energy that keeps us alert and alive and aware.

We were discussing Shangri-la at breakfast this morning—the dream place, the place where everything is exactly the way you want it; your idea of what the ultimate place would be. But I think Shangri-la is sometimes overstressed. We really want too much to find *the* place. We want to find the ultimate method of enlightenment—whether it's yoga or zen or t'ai chi or sufi or whatever. When you begin to think that anything is *the* thing then you really limit yourself. There's no such thing as *the* method.

Last night was very revealing to me. We were doing folk-dancing and I heard familiar music. I started dancing and I thought "Oh yes, I know it, I know it." When everybody was still going this way, I switched directions because I was thinking ahead—and I hit the lady next to me right on the teeth. After that I stopped thinking and began to relax into the music and I got the rest of the dance in the right sequence. When we finished dancing I went over to the lady and apologized, saying "I'm sorry I lost my sense of t'ai chi." She said, "Oh I guess it's O.K.—even professional people make mistakes. That makes me feel good." I said, "Professional people make *more* mistakes." In fact, the only way to become a professional is to make a lot of glorious, beautiful, huge mistakes. How do you learn anything without making mistakes? You make mistakes in order to find a way to do it. T'ai chi is only *a* way. A way is not *the* way. It's not the perfect way. I would never go around and tell you that this is *it*, that "I have found t'ai chi ch'uan is the ultimate, most perfect thing you can ever do

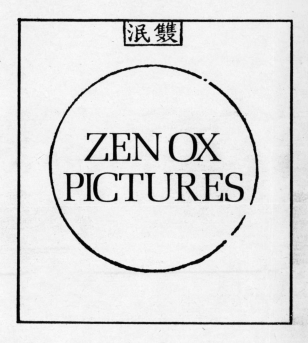

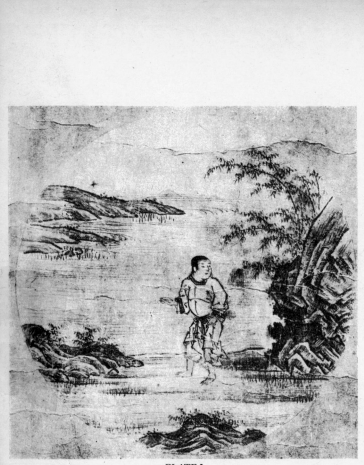

PLATE I.

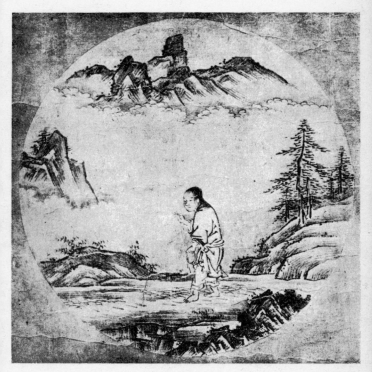

PLATE II.

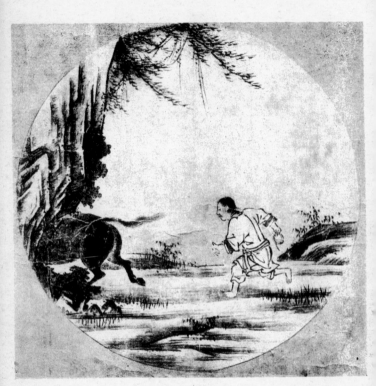

PLATE III.

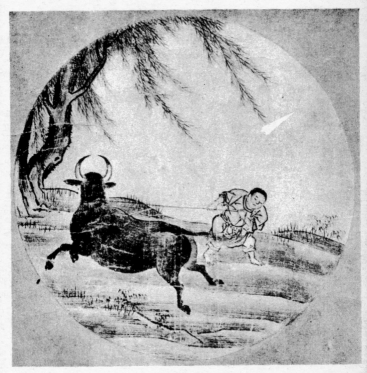

PLATE IV.

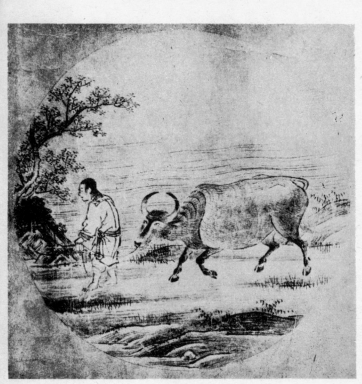

PLATE V.

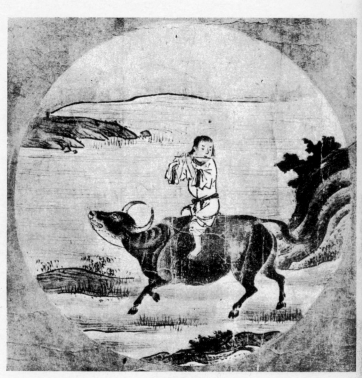

PLATE VI.

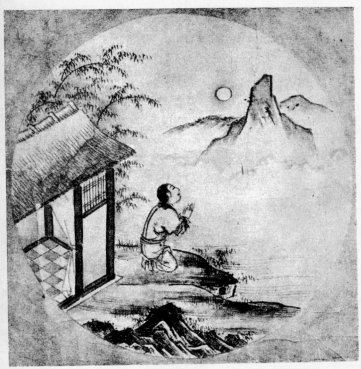

PLATE VII.

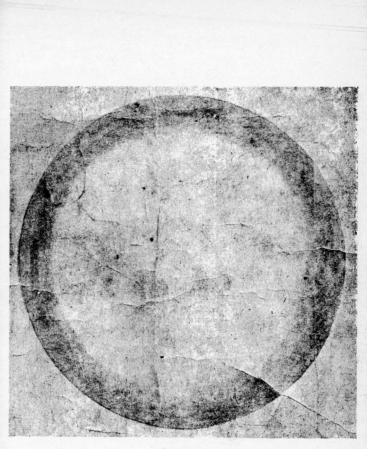

PLATE VIII.

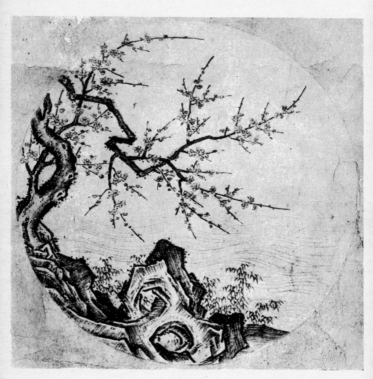

PLATE IX.

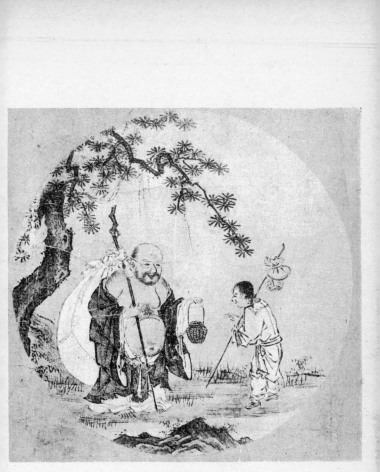

PLATE X.

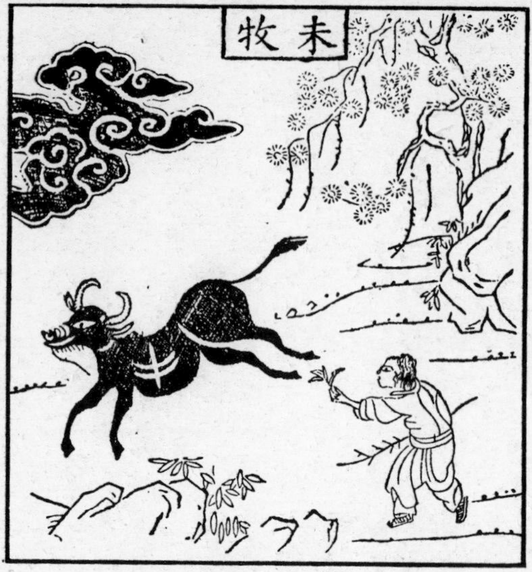

PLATE XI.

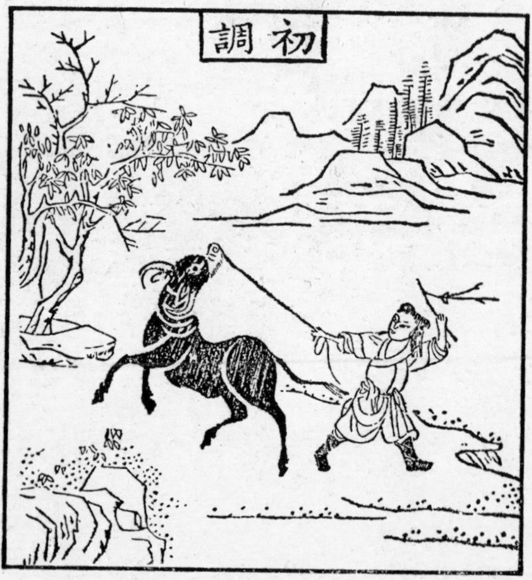

PLATE XII.

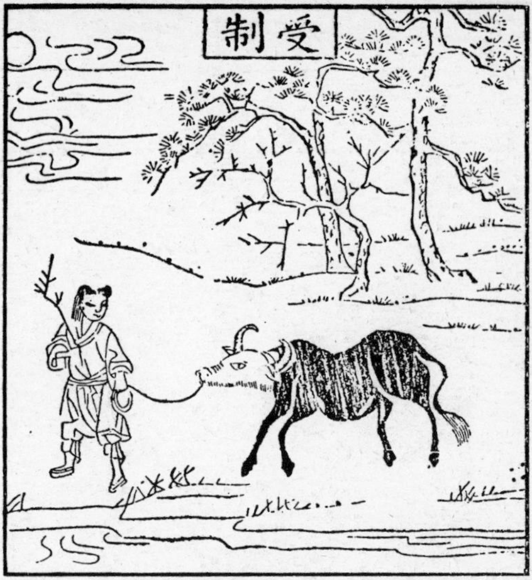

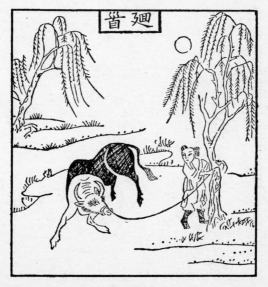

制受

PLATE XIII.

首廻

PLATE XIV.

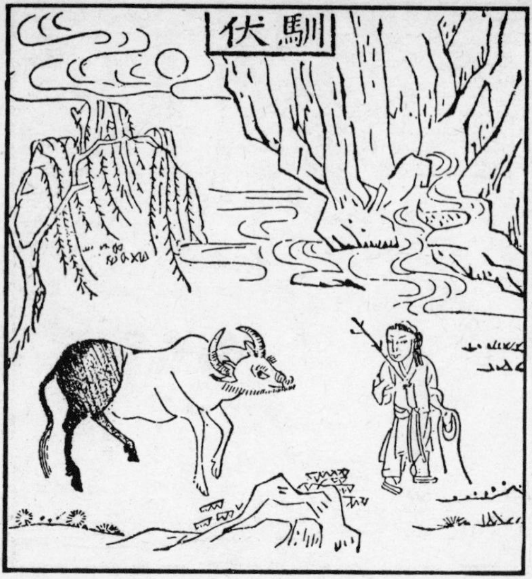

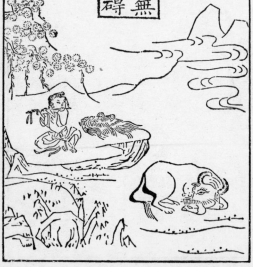

PLATE XV.

PLATE XVI.

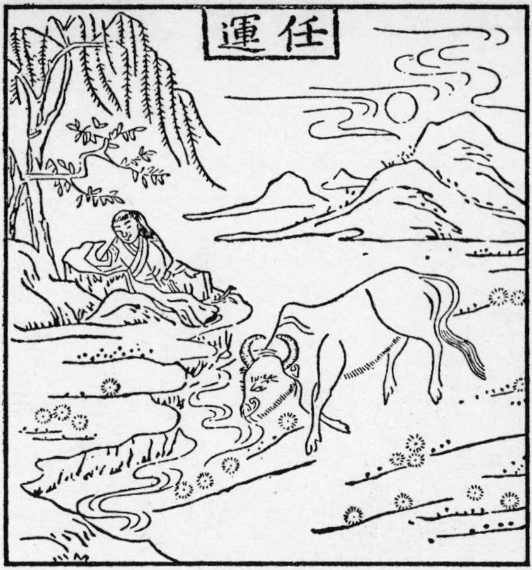

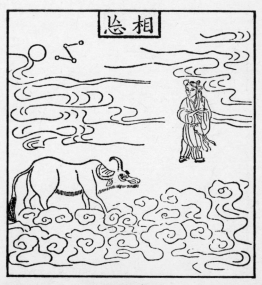

任運

PLATE XVII.

相忘

PLATE XVIII.

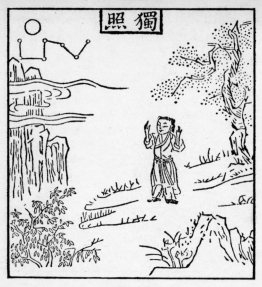

PLATE XIX.

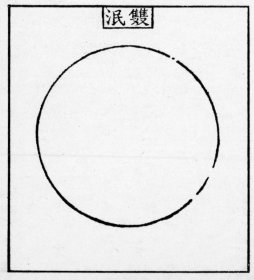

PLATE XX.

for your body." There's no such thing. It doesn't make *me* perfect. Just because I practice t'ai chi doesn't mean that I can do everything well. Everything still presents a challenge to me.

The only way your body can be completely flowing is in practicing t'ai chi the natural way. If you allow the body to go and fulfill its curve and its own strength, then no extra tension will build. But we know very well that none of us will ever be able to completely flow through—totally undistracted by physical, mental and other environmental energies. You do react, you do stop short and do things that interrupt the movement. Therefore the new stress, the new tension comes in. T'ai chi can help you to recognize that and then to release it all over again each time. That's why you take time to begin moving in the morning. In the early morning you're not in a rush to get anywhere, and there is enough time to let go for a while. However far you can let your body and your thinking go, let it, and then you're more ready to be receptive to events. That's all. Most of us are very impressionable and easily persuaded. I often hear people say, "He is my guru. Come, meet my guru," or "This is the book, you gotta read this book." If you get stuck with one way, then you have real problems. If you don't get stuck, you can flow out of it and go through it; it becomes you and disappears.

Someone was asking, "Al, what's the difference between your t'ai chi and my t'ai chi?" I said, "The difference is, I'm I and you're you, and we are somewhat different." The Al Huang today doesn't even know Al Huang yesterday or Al Huang tomorrow. Al Huang only knows Al Huang *now*. And I'm only able to perceive and listen and live and be with all of you now.

I think we reach a common ground when we get to the point of realizing we don't know anything. Then we can begin all over again together. T'ai chi does this for us—suddenly, we don't know anything. When you begin to practice t'ai chi, you begin exactly the same way, by emptying yourself. You begin your new t'ai chi each day, each time. You don't have to be reminded that you should connect this muscle with that muscle with that much energy because the electromyogram has indicated that's just right. Yesterday we were talking about this device that measures muscle movements. I said, "Oh, wonderful, now I know how to present a New York concert. I won't have to spend months and years to train my dancers. All I have to do is get a computer tape to program the muscle concert in New York. No critic will dare say anything negative because I will have all the statistics on my side."

One of the nice things about working in the arts is that they don't deal with the measurable, countable parts of the human existence. The things that really tie us together as human beings, as people, are the things that we really have no visible means or approachable way of measuring. Maybe we find a new way of expressing a feeling, a new way of saying, a new way of doing, but most of the time we are repeating the same old thing. Life *is* this way. Every morning begins the same but develops differently. And t'ai chi begins the same, but it's always different.

Now I would like to establish that mutual ground again and then work on variations. First I want to work in a circular moving pattern, so let's get up and join our hands in a circle. I love circles. Even when you work alone, you should feel the connection of this circle. Let's help each other to get the body to feel the fluidity. Release your tensions by swaying with everybody's flow. Take a few minutes to just sense your own energy level, your position, your tightness, whatever you feel now. If you've been listening too hard and the tension is getting you down, think of release. As your body begins to free itself, work from the center, and let the energy from your center begin to move your torso slightly.

Undulate your spine and let your hips come into this movement. Let your torso bend and twist. If you move your body around too much, then you can really feel why you need that center to come back to. We tend to use our extremities too much. We see with our eyeballs popping out. We reach with our hands without feeling the connection of the movement with our center.

While still holding hands, get your whole body moving. Look around the circle from one person to the next and let your vision connect with your body. Sense the transmission of movement through your hands. Now you can close your eyes and still feel this connection and movement.

The feet are moving now, so let's travel a bit around the circle. Experience the feeling of how you cross your legs and change your position while maintaining that center. Do you have to think which leg comes first, or can you let the spine pivot and let the leg follow naturally? If your arms are getting tired from holding your muscles, let them droop a little bit.

Now slow down and drop hands. Mill around and exchange places with someone directly opposite you in the circle. Do this in a playful way. Don't do it directly. You can have all kinds of nice distractions on the way—perhaps dancing with several people. Don't get there too efficiently or fast, or you will have to stand around and wait. Efficiency creates a lot of time, and if you don't know what to do with it, it creates boredom and misery. It's nice to get somewhere, but don't ignore what's happening on the way. Sometimes it's much more interesting than your goal. The shortest distance between two points is a straight line. That's the efficient way to solve the problem. But what next? Maybe I'll get bored with all the time I saved. Maybe I'd rather have fun along the way. So I start moving and looping and I enjoy the process of getting there. The end result of this is very different than just going straight across. This is what the *process* is all about.

What we are doing is a good example of the idea of form in t'ai chi. Changing places is the form or structure. What happens *within* the form is what you create for yourself in the process of doing it. When you really learn t'ai chi, it's not just a set of positions everyone can recognize exactly. What happens *in between* is the real creative process.

The next time you begin to move toward the person opposite you, be open to the whole group, ready to find a new place as the circle alters. You may find that the person you expected to change places with has already changed with someone else.

We've been working a lot on your awareness of what's around you as you move. People bump into us all the time. This morning at breakfast it happened to me twice. The first time, I was very successful in flowing out. The second time, the force came so abruptly that my cereal splashed all over my jacket. This same clash would happen if we all suddenly rushed directly toward the person opposite us without paying any attention to anyone else. If you move with awareness of your surroundings, then you don't clash or collide. In a tiny little room like this, you might think you can't dance very much. But the past few nights very few people have been hitting each other, even with very fancy big swinging movements.

When I was a child we used to go around and push each other behind the knees and make the legs collapse. Most children take it as a game and laugh about it and enjoy it. When we got a little older we got very indignant if someone did it to us—which only made it more fun to do. Pretty soon everyone was walking around with stiff, rigid legs to be safe. Let's try returning to the young child's view of this. Walk around and push in behind each other's knees and respond by yielding to the push. Instead of resisting, let your knees be resilient. Bounce down and then gently straighten up again. Imagine that your legs have big springs and shock absorbers so that you can give in easily instead of being toppled or having to stand rigidly to resist the push.

When any outside energy comes to you, when the force literally pushes towards you and against you, instead of rejecting and resisting, *receive* it and bring it back down into your center. Then, if it becomes unbearable, all you have to do is pivot your body and spin out of it. You become like a bouncing ball on top of the water—when it is pushed, it bounces out, the circle rounds it off. There's no need to worry about being pushed under, pushed aside, or not being able to receive the shock. Shock is a result of your own resistance to an external force. When you allow this force to come to you and spin around with you, you can have fun with it. This is an example of the value of being vulnerable, of not being afraid to be flexible, and open to receive.

Do this now, as you're walking around. Push each other a little and try to enjoy being shoved. Let yourself be vulnerable and take in the energy when you bump into someone. Let each push give you a ride as you spin off away from the person who bumped into you. There's no need to fight the energy—it comes to you and you go with it. There's no work involved, so just have fun. Every once in a while you may get a force which is a little vicious and catches you off guard. But even then, if you allow the rebound to happen, it will just send you into a new spin without shock or concussion. There is no way to attack something that rolls away like a beach ball.

If you look for a safe spot to hang on to and you don't want to move, you refuse to budge—then if someone pushes you around you feel defeated, rejected, like you are being removed from your security. But if you don't try to hang onto anything, you can move with a sense of carrying your security with you. Wherever you are, you have your base. Wherever you go, you have your sense of yourself. You don't have to worry about "How to go; where to go? Is it best to go that way or the other way?" You just go with the energy and have yourself a spin. You flow with that energy and play with it.

Sometimes we worry about losing what we have gained. We think of ourselves as having a stable state, a safe place. We think of ourselves as already *there*, and we resist anything new. But if we don't have anything to hang onto and protect, then we receive much more readily. We are not as defensive and tense about letting whatever happens around us come to us.

Now let's do some more t'ui sho, which is one of the best ways of getting more of this sense of yielding into your body. It helps you to discover how you are disrupting the flow with tension and helps you to work through these tense areas. Find a partner about your height, but don't join hands yet. Stand opposite each other, slightly apart, and make a half circle of space in front of you with your arms. Now walk toward each other until you complete your half-circle with your partner's half-circle. This kind of coming together is more t'ai chi, because you have to move through the empty space until the two halves become one as you touch fingertips.

Feel your mutual base now. Open your base a little wider and settle down into it. Relax your elbows and shoulders and imagine that the space beneath your arms is a moving surface that supports them. Sway and curve a little and let your arms move together. Allow the energy to flow through your arms, through your partner's body and then return back where you pick it up again. Literally think of your energy transmitted through your right arm into your partner's left arm, across his back and through his right arm. This energy comes back to your left hand and circles across your own body and is then transmitted out again. T'ui sho should be an ongoing, never-ending process of energy giving and receiving.

Now release your partner and step back. When you move forward again, join right hands to make a shared S-shape. Now bring your left hand up to touch your partner's right elbow. Together you have made a yin/yang symbol with your arms, the t'ai chi circle divided by an S-shaped line. It shows that the energy of one side is always flowing into the other. One side is the white fish and one side is the black fish, depending on who is pushing and who is receiving at the moment.

Now rotate your wrists and let a small circular

movement develop right in the center of the circle, where your right hands are joined. Relax your right elbows and let them sink. Use your partner's supporting left hand under your elbow to help you to keep your arm up without holding and tensing. Allow your body to move forward and back in the same circular motion as your hands, revolving around your spine/center. The gentle pushing gesture of the palm is yang, and the soft scooping-back gesture is yin. You push energy toward your partner, and then gather it back toward you. Keep your wrist relaxed and resilient, so that it can revolve easily as it circles.

As your hand pushes out it's an attacking movement, and as it scoops in, it's a shielding movement. Actually feel the sensation in the part of your body that is sending or receiving energy. Feel the palm of your hand as you push out, and the outside of your arm that receives the energy of your partner's push. Also feel the inside of your arm and the protected circle of space between your shielding arm and your body.

If you step together around the circle that you have created between your arms, this will help you to let go of tension. Your right foot should be near the center of the circle, as you move counterclockwise around that circle. This center is a constant point to return to. When you think of the space underneath you supporting you, and this pivoting point, you can begin to forget the work of the arms and become more relaxed. If your feet are nailed down, you can't adjust to receive a new return of energy. Sink into your base so you can feel the spine connecting into the ground, with energy coming up easily through your back into your upper body. Let the whole body be open, so that even the back of your heel can feel the hand connection. Close your eyes for a while to help you focus on the feeling of the movement.

Now make the circle a little bigger as you put more energy into your movement. As the circle gets bigger you have to expand the curve of the energy, and you have to move back farther to receive your partner's energy. Since you can't go straight back, you have to go to one side. If you do a very small circle with your hands, you will find you have enough range to just go straight back and forth on your base. But when the circle gets bigger you may try to bend your back and lean backwards. This is very unwise because then you become really unbalanced. But if you turn toward your open side, then you can let the energy go past you by pivoting your spine while keeping it straight.

Remember that when I say to keep a straight, upright spine, I don't mean a rigid, tense spine. Your spine becomes straight by *allowing* it, not by tensing it or holding it. The t'ai chi spine is a floating, extending line—growing upward and rooting downward. When you feel tightness in your spine, release it and let it move, and then let it return to this basic center of a straight, upright line. Let your spine feel like bamboo weighed down by snow or being bent by the wind, that bounces back when the force is removed. Every time you let your spine go, it springs back to that easy supple straightness. If you are rigid and brittle, then you cannot withstand the weight, and you will break and snap. Bodies must be elastic, curving, resilient.

Feel how your partner responds to your movement and how you respond to his. Sense it without trying to manipulate each other. If you feel your partner too strong, then yield: go along with his yang. As you go with the yang, the force of yang will become yin. If you try to fight the yang, you will have two yang forces and you will collide. That's the beginning of conflict. If you begin to drive each other around, you won't enjoy the circle. It will become very square and you will get stuck in the many corners. If you get unbalanced, slow down until you can easily match up with each other with a minimum of holding, supporting energy.

Now get a little closer to each other so that your supported elbows are practically touching and feel very much connected with your spine. Your forearms are almost vertical, like the center of a flower that is growing up between you. Move even closer to your partner until your knees touch and you can feel them circling together in the same way your wrists are circling. If your kneecaps are bumping, this shows that the motion of your wrists is isolated and not carried throughout your body. I see that some of you are rocking straight back and forward instead of around in a circle. If I put a white dot on your kneecap, on your shoulders, or anywhere else on your body, it should be making a circle when viewed from above. Every part of your body must go with that circular motion. Most of you tend to compensate unevenly. If your hips are moving in a circle and your knees are going forward and back, you're not consistent and then these different movements will clash. Your whole body must respond and be connected to your moving contact with your partner.

Now very slowly move back from your partner and make the circle a little bigger without tensing up and holding the elbow. Maintain that easy feeling of your supported elbow, and the natural rotation of your wrists as your hand moves in a circle in contact with your partner. When you feel tension, *give in* to it instead of fighting it: say "yes" to it, instead of "no." What tenses you up is the yang energy of intention, trying too hard. Let the yielding yin energy come in more.

T'ui sho helps you to get to know your own body by your partner's reflection of you. The benefits only come through long practice. Just keep practicing, without worrying about "Am I getting better?" You know when you still have tension in the body because you can sense the tired muscles, trying to *do* instead of letting-be. The more you worry about these things, the harder it is to get rid of the tensions. When you begin to feel comfortable in the upper body, pay attention to the feeling of the movement of the lower body—the base and the sequential details of the movement of the feet and legs.

Look out at the rain on the deck today. Watch

how each drop of rain makes a pinpoint contact in the puddles, and then an expanding circle that settles and disappears as it gently overlaps with other circles. This is very much the feeling of t'ai chi. Every one of the movements, every part of the form is like a clear circle in the water. The circles are temporary. Each movement is like a changing, overlapping, disappearing pattern of circles. See how each new circle returns to the clear, calm, open surface again.

Clench your fist, and then let it open. Let the tight energy open up and dissolve within your hand, like the expanding circle of the raindrop in the puddle. You cannot last very long doing this clenching. If most of your energy goes into clenching your fist, you will soon have very little left. Now release this fist you have been clenching and feel the tingling in your hand as the natural circulation returns. Feel the energy inside. Let your thumb lightly touch your fingers as if you are gently holding something small in your hand. In t'ai chi we call this "the empty fist."

Most people think of a clenched fist as a symbol of strength. "I'm strong because I have a very strong fist, I can beat you up. I can break the board in half. I can break the brick." But there's a big difference between energy and strength. Energy is not that external expression of a heavy, clenched, straining fist. Nor is it a weak, useless fist. The t'ai chi fist is right in the middle, neither totally clenched nor completely limp. It's an empty, moving, ready fist.

Now use this empty fist to punch slowly into your other palm. As you punch into it, let this palm cover the fist as if it were a piece of cloth. Let the left palm encircle the empty fist to complete the gesture of covering. When the cloth and fist become one, your punching energy is unified. Now form a bowl with both hands, and draw the energy back into your tant'ien. Then push the ch'i back out, and around, and over you.

Let your arms open up as if you are embracing the whole world in front of you. This curve is the beginning of a motif called Embrace Tiger. Then let your arms curve downward and inward and scoop up all this space. Your arms cross low in front of you as you lift this energy. Keep your spine straight and settle into your base with knees bent. Keep lifting this energy up to chest-level. Now let your elbows sink and let your wrists rotate inward until you are gently settling all this energy downward into your tant'ien. We call this settling back to the simple beginning stance, Return to Mountain.

Embrace Tiger, Return to Mountain is a nice circular motif to warm up with. It's also a good movement to use to increase your awareness of the coordination of your breathing with the movement. From the beginning standing position, just let your arms float up sideways as you inhale. When your arms reach about shoulder height settle into your base as your arms scoop downward and inward. Exhale as you gather in the space, and then inhale as you scoop it up and begin to lift. When your arms turn and push downward towards the tant'ien you exhale again.

Usually every time there is a rise in the body, you inhale; and every time the body sinks, you breathe out. As you extend the body and reach out you breathe in, and as you return to center, air moves out. It's like a balloon: As your body sinks and pulls in, air goes out, and as it rises and expands, air comes in. Don't make a particular point to start breathing out or in. There is no one place for breathing out or in, and no exact place where you change. Also, the practice of t'ai chi tends to eliminate the idea of an in/out duality. You are the union of both as you practice t'ai chi. You are breathing all around, all over. As you do t'ai chi it's not up or down only. It's up . . . down, downuuuup down up up up downdown up—wave follows wave follows wave. You notice that air comes in somewhere in the curve, but you can't plan it. The moment you try to plan it, you break the continuous curve into segments.

When your breathing feels right to you, without straining or thinking, then its fine. Often in the morning when we begin t'ai chi, we practice breathing naturally with the rise and fall as in this Tiger/Mountain movement. This is the only time that you can really consciously work on the breathing. The minute you begin to move laterally it's more than just this *or* this, and that—it's *everything*, so your breathing has to flow with the movement. When you really get into t'ai chi, you are suspended in the center, and everything simply happens and unfolds around you.

V

I don't know if there are any weary bones and sore muscles in the group, but I see many pairs of shining eyes, maybe from the dancing last night or perhaps from just generally feeling good in the body. I like the way we begin this morning, sitting quietly together in a circle, looking and smiling at each other and sensing ourselves together as a group. I like talking with you at the breakfast table and at night after our session about what's happening. This is how I keep in touch with how we're doing.

This morning somebody mentioned that yesterday's afternoon session went a little too fast. I was glad to hear that comment. I feel a certain obligation as leader, and sometimes my anxiety makes me rush a little. But I also know that if I can get you into a state of motion, you will pick up the ideas and movements much more easily. If I ask you to stand still and listen, then you will all freeze. But if you are already moving, then when another motion comes to you, you just flow into it and the t'ai chi works for you immediately. Last night you were moving beautifully. But if any time during the session you really are involved in one movement, and I push you into another one, tell me to slow down. This will help me to relieve my anxiety of trying to complete the circle too soon.

I want to say a few things about the dancing last night. For me dance is not a form or shape that you categorize. Dancing is a state of true awareness of your body movement. When you are able to allow the body to be in touch with that flow, then you are dancing. The big difficulty is usually the comparing and judging that goes on in your mind. Instead of just letting movement happen, you try to be very careful to make beautiful movements and not make ugly ones, so you freeze up and become rigid and awkward.

Last night, in the beginning there were only a few people dancing. This tends to put you in a position of being watched, and that puts a burden on you. You see someone else doing something fantastic and you begin to compare it to your own movement. If you try to copy his movement, you begin forcing yourself from the outside.

But if you see someone else moving and you pay attention to your own responses to his movement, then you can move out of your own center. Then you can feel excitement and movement in your body and allow it to emerge and grow and develop without comparing it or judging it. True dancing is letting your awareness flow into movement. Be aware of what is happening around you and pick up and use each other's energy. Dance with each other, and respond to each other's movements and gestures. Make connections. This is the kind of dancing that I find most fulfilling.

But don't just cling together and never let go, thinking that you are dancing together. If you are both just repeating a set pattern over and over again you might as well be dancing robots. But if you are allowing your own movement to develop and at the same time are aware of other people's curves and energies, then you are always open and aware of dancing with each other. This is dancing at its most open, full range. But it must be *your* range, your own openness, your own spontaneity, your turns, your control, your connection, your unity in the body. Utilize the t'ai chi curve, so that every extension of energy returns to you and keeps you moving without getting tired. You keep sending energy out and it always returns to you without getting lost. You send it out to that person in front of you; he sends it back, and you send it over to another, and then it comes back to you again.

One of the wonderful things about the so-called "now" social dancing is that it has a certain spontaneity of letting go. The only problem is that most of the time it's a *throwing* of energy, which doesn't return, so people get exhausted. Many young people have a lot of frustration and energy that they want to get rid of. But as we get older we don't really want to get rid of energy: We want to utilize it; we want to preserve it. The understanding of t'ai chi in your body helps you to release energy with the feeling of being able to bring it back in a curve and re-use it. "Dancing cheek to cheek" may be one way of expressing togetherness, but I think you can be just as close to each other dancing apart, as long as you continue to relate to each other. There is no need to match movement like a mirror-image, or follow each other like a shadow. This is why when we practice together, I do not insist on your following me exactly, giving us the look of a T'ai Chi Squad. Observers may compliment you on your form because you can do it exactly the way your master does it. But they don't realize that out of the corner of your eye you have been following like mad, and you never really did it yourself!

When I was a child we used to get up every morning and go to the t'ai chi master and just breathe and practice the beginning arm-rising. The master would never let us do more than just this, for months. If I ask you all here to do even six days of this, you're going to quit and ask for a refund! What kept me going as a child was noticing what was happening. One cold morning, maybe it's playing with my steaming breath. If it's early, there's dew drops on the bamboo leaves. Another morning there's a frog hopping, or birds flying. If you are not observant, then *of course* you get bored.

Things change: it's never the same. The constant always relates to the changes. If we wear horseblinders then we miss the fun of life. T'ai chi is the understanding of how to be content with your constant, so you are able to perceive the changes. T'ai chi is awareness, t'ai chi is coming back to center so you can open up and perceive and flow.

Last night we had some new people come into the group, people who were not familiar with what we have been doing. At first our own group clung onto its familiar unity and became stronger, but separate from the new people. Then as each of us got more centered we pulled the new people in with us to become one group again. I think everybody got into the flow at least part of the time.

We had a wide range of willingness and openness and honesty in this new group. But how do we compare these different qualities? Is someone standing by the door, just allowing his shoulders to move a little, any better or worse than the man kicking his legs very high? Who is honest and who is willing? Maybe both are, or maybe both aren't. The man who is kicking his legs high might be straining to show off, while the man at the door might be really aware and in tune with his body and what's happening around him. So there's no comparison, they are just two different things.

By comparing, you detach yourself from the flow of what's happening in you and around you and become preoccupied with evaluating and judging, thinking and worrying. If you are dancing and you see someone watching you, you may get self-conscious. Instead of separating yourself from the watcher, you can include him in your movement space. Both you and the watcher will feel more comfortable when you are connecting, your movement flowing around his stillness. Maybe he will receive some of your energy and begin moving with you. Whether he dances with you or not, you will be connected with him. You can both allow your own movement to happen without ignoring or interfering with each other.

Last night many beautiful things happened. Steve really got going and was swooping in and out of the group. For such a big person, he was very thin moving around so fast in such a dense group of people. Natalie and I were doing shoulder-dancing for a while. Our shoulder joints seemed to melt together. Roger and Alberta had a marvelous spin going that went on and on and on. Dannelle said to me that by dancing, by allowing herself to be, she realized what she had absorbed during the past few days. She did not consciously think, "Ah, today I learned this and that; I gained this much." You do not do it step by step that way, by adding on coatings of varnish, or new paint. When learning *becomes* you, then it appears as you need it, when you are being you. Sometimes true learning surprises you when it emerges. This is what we call wu wei—doing by not doing, doing by allowing to happen. But it takes both you and the environment, the sensitivity to both yourself and to the group, to create that confidence. It's not something that you can boast about—"I'm confident, I'm secure, look how good I am." If you're really secure, you don't have to do anything about it. It will emerge in your own body.

Now we can look back on last night and realize that it is a memory of the past. For some people maybe this is one of the highlights of their lives. Others maybe never really got with it. Either way it is fine; that was that experience. Don't expect it to happen again just like that. It won't. Nothing will be the same if you begin to compare everything with what happened last night. You will be separating yourself from your experience and rejecting everything because it isn't the way you expect it to be. But if you allow yourself to absorb an experience like last night, then you will learn from it and then the next time you begin to dance you will have more awareness. By dance I mean not only just when you move with music, but also the flow in your walk between here and your cabin, and when you go to get coffee in the busy dining room.

It's a joy to see the many beautiful, subtle, softenings of your bodies that happen throughout the day. That's true dancing. There are always people who

have had more training and can get their legs higher.
People who have natural agility often tend to show
off quite a bit. I know because I used to be a big
show-off. It's still easy for me to fall back into that
bad habit of trying to be something "special" instead
of just being what I am at the moment. We all tend
to want to learn something so we can show off one
way or the other. You must admit you like to do things
you know you can do pretty well.

When you move with music or with any kind of
rhythm, the important thing is to make the rhythm a
part of you and relate to that rhythm, so you are
working *with* the musicians. You do not dance *to*
music, you dance *within* the music. This is why I
asked the musicians to play in the middle of the room,
so we could dance around them. We can use the
magic circle again to feel that there is not an opposition: "They are *there, playing* sound; we are *here,
receiving* sound." As they began to warm up their
sound, there was the sound within ourselves corre-
sponding to it. And then by the time we felt our sound
and their sound becoming one, we were dancing.

The musicians said they liked the feeling of being
in the middle of it, instead of having people watch
them perform, but not really *with* them. I understand
this, because when I dance on the stage there are the
footlights, and the people all sitting there watching.
In the west, we go to a theater to sit in a comfortable
chair and look up on the stage to see a performer
doing something special. This is the so-called "esthetic
distance" in theater, the "fourth wall" situation. It's
as if you have permission to peek through a keyhole
as long as it's in the theater. But you know that what
you see is not real; it's just play-acting. If an actor on
stage dies, you can appreciate it yet remain comfort-
ably apart.

In the east, we don't make a special point of em-
phasizing this distance. If an actor dies on stage, he
will go through all the motions of dying and then just
get up and walk off—and you accept that. An actor
will be singing his aria and in the midst of it a prop

man will come in to give him a cup of tea. The actor simply lifts his wide sleeve to cover his mouth as he drinks his tea. Then he gives the cup back to the prop man and continues on with the song.

This is much more honest and spontaneous than most of us here are accustomed to. In contrast to the solemn atmosphere of most western theater, Chinese theater is fun and casual. Behind every seat in the audience there is a tea cup. Hawkers keep coming around to sell you tea and food. Hot towels are passed around to keep you awake. People eat lunch and crack watermelon seeds, while children run around and drape themselves over the edge of the stage. It's more of a living, give-and-take situation. There's no set time for applause. When actors do well, the audience sings along with the actors and gets all excited. When they don't do well, they boo and throw things on the stage. All the Chinese plays have been handed down for centuries. Everybody knows exactly what will happen. There are no mysterious endings. The stories depicted are fantastic and bigger than life. They are so familiar to both the audience and the actors that each must recreate the essence each time and let the moment come to life. No one pretends that it never happened before. It's an acceptance that there's really nothing new under the sun. There's no egotism from the actor about "I invented this," or from the audience that "I perceive this like nobody else."

I love to observe a group of fine musicians working together. Those of you who enjoy jazz know that jazz musicians understand t'ai chi; they really know how to improvise together. They really talk back and forth with their music. In the Chinese theater the musicians and the performers are also right in tune with each other. The percussionists follow the movements and gestures of the actors very closely and make them audible. They breathe with each other.

In this country, if a ballet has live music, the conductor will conduct, and the dancers will try to follow the music. The dancers have usually been rehearsing with tapes so they know how many measures they must dance to. But every once in a while they'll get a new conductor without enough time to rehearse. They'll find the tempo changed and the result is ludicrous because they can't adjust. This is the problem you run into when you *think* you have a common denominator, some solid reference point. You take it for granted, and when you lose it it's a disaster. In oriental theater there's no such thing as exact, set timing. There is no music or movement notation you can write down. The Chinese actor learns his roles by singing with his movements. This way the timing of the singing comes out of the movement timing. When they dig it and do it fully, the timing becomes intrinsic.

Most people who come to a music session just listen and get into their own trance. I get very depressed when I see a room full of introspective people, because the lack of connection develops alienation. We should open ourselves to the music, so that by the end we will feel like we have really experienced what's happened around us.

One thing I noticed last night is that it was easy for most of us to stick exactly with the beat of the musicians, but pretty difficult for us to ride on it freely. What is rhythm? Each one of us has a slightly different rhythm. There's a certain rhythm about this place. It's a flow. It's a feeling of how you flow with something else. Sometimes we say the rhythm of life. It's not just a beat or trying to hit it exactly. There is no need to get stuck with the pulse. Your own rhythm can go on top of it, or underneath, or in and out of it. But this interweaving with the music is more difficult. It's like the t'ai chi transition that continues to flow and doesn't stop. You can' hit each beat; you must feel the energy changing all the time or you lose the constant. When the drummer is playing, even though he's marking each beat, he feels the constant sound connection. And this is why good musicians end beautifully when they play together. They flow to a tail that curves.

Some of you have talked about learning a short

form of t'ai chi, which has certain transitional motifs eliminated. The reason for certain repetitions is to help you flow within the form—to ride over it without thinking. When these repetitions are cut out, some of the transitions may become awkward. When different movements are jammed together, the sequence loses some of its smoothness.

When you first begin to practice, you keep thinking, "This follows that—after this, it's this and then that." It's still a mental process that you have to suffer through until you get beyond the programming. After you practice for a while, the in-between movements become just as important.

The form just gives you a way of flowing through. It's a passing thing: it's not a set thing. If a photographer wants to take a picture, you don't really know when to tell him to take it. You can't say, "Now, this is it." We have a tendency, visually, to find the extremes—the length and the depth of things. In t'ai chi we do not stress length as a positive—tallness is not better than shortness, roundness is not better than thinness. All the contrasting factors must be melted together.

Many people ask me, "Do you use music for your t'ai chi? What kind do you use?" and I say, "It depends on what kind of music is happening at the time." Usually when I think of t'ai chi music I think of nature's sounds. This is the sound you can always depend on and use to move in contact with your surroundings—raindrops, ocean, traffic sounds, airplanes, bird songs, leaves rustling. I was given a tape of the sounds of the San Diego Zoo at five o'clock in the morning. It's filled with the sounds of baboons yawning, hornbills waking up, and gibbons carrying on a heated conversation. Suddenly you hear the "putt-putt-putt" of a motor-driven tree-trimmer.

You use the *available* sound. For instance, we're in Big Sur now. Open up to the sound of the ocean, the muffled sound of the fog in the morning, the sound that is happening now. It would be a big joke on ourselves if I played a tape of the ocean here. When we were having coffee, somebody said, "Have you seen the cartoon of the little boy watching the snow falling on TV, while snow is falling outside the window?" We have to recognize that folly in ourselves. Why do we gather around and talk about nature when nature is all around us? If we don't feel it, if we don't allow nature to happen to us as a self-learning experience, it won't do any good to talk about it.

Sometimes we chant when we practice t'ai chi to extend the element of the one continuous flow of energy. We use what we have, which is our voice. A lot of people chant Om. Some people have mystical or religious reasons for choosing Om, but for me it's simply a nice flowing sound. You form that round shape with your mouth and you allow the sound to come through. When I was a child, we used to chant "na mu o me to fo" which is a Chinese version of a Buddhist chant. It's arbitrary. It's just one variation of a general flowing sound that you can really feel coming out from your center.

The only objection to music with t'ai chi would be if it was heavily structured. It would be odd to do t'ai chi with three/four time, because the heavy emphasis on the first beat would give a pendulum-like quality to your movement. The up-down side-to-side swinging would be overemphasized and the rest of the movement would be lost. If we tried four/four time we'd keep hitting the beat, and the movements would look like the static pictures of each t'ai chi position" in so many instruction books. It would look like everybody was counting a structured beat. Some of us were sitting at the breakfast table observing a few people practicing t'ai chi on the deck. I heard the comment, "They must be counting." They may not have been counting, but their movement did give a definite impression of a structured beat. We must not *see* that when you practice t'ai chi, even though it's an underlying thing. It's like the drum beat. If you keep up with the sound of every beat, you will be tense and spastic. If the drummer counts everything he beats, his wrists will get very tired because each count will be a separate need for new energy.

Several summers ago I had a chance to work with a group of musicians in La Jolla. Pauline Oliveros and some of her ♀ ensemble had attended several of my t'ai chi workshops and noticed how their own group worked together in a similar way. Since then we have shared many seminars and concerts together, exploring the t'ai chi sound. We sit and breathe, and allow things to happen. Most of the time we begin simply, with our voices chanting om or whatever sound comes freely. We let the one-note sound come through, the one-note sound that is also a million sounds. Within that one sound we can hear all sounds. The instruments we most often use, besides voice, are winds, strings, even an accordion—any instruments which are able to sustain notes.

Let's try this. Sit in an easy cross-legged position. The important thing is to allow this space in front of you to be open. If you are bending over too much you will have tightness here in front. Really feel the tant'ien—the diaphragm or the lower abdominal area —and keep it open.

Now recall the circular breathing that we did earlier. Just observe the natural flow of your breathing. Don't push the air out by force or suck it in by will. Just allow that organic process to take place.

If you think "When do I begin to use my vocal cords?" then you have already stopped flowing. Your voice will tighten and your breathing will become irregular. But if you just let the flow of your breathing happen, then the sound from within you will spontaneously emerge as an audible note.

In chanting, the sound of your voice comes out as an extension of you, not as a separate part of you. You don't hear it as a separate thing. You don't say, "Oh, that's a nice tone, I like that." It's a tone that grows out of you. I've heard a lot of chanting. Sometimes people really get very carried away with the beautiful sounds they make. But in the best chanting sessions I have been in, we allowed openness all over —not just a vocal openness. It's as if there is openness even in the pores of your body, and the sound grows out of you. You make a total body sound, and everybody's sound becomes yours.

Very often we think of music that has a recognizable melody, or a clear rhythmical pattern. When you hear something relatively un-metered and without all that fluctuation, you can get bored easily. But if you really hear it and sing along with it and chant with it, and you become it and move with it, then the one-note sound becomes a million sounds. When totally involved, musicians can go on for hours with the same kind of sound without stopping, because they are *inside* the sound.

Erik Satie has a very short piece that is supposed to be repeated three hundred times when it is performed. It was played in New York by several pianists who alternated and kept repeating the piece. I think they sold tickets for about eight dollars and the longer you stayed, the more refund you got back. The whole thing lasted about twelve hours. It's a matter of involvement: if you really get involved, time is relative. What is a lifetime? What is an instant?

The best sound for t'ai chi is really that open silence inside, that allows the sounds around you to come in. If you are at Big Sur, it's the ocean; in the mountains, it's the mountain sounds. If you are doing t'ai chi in the subway, it's something else.

Once I was on a lurching, jerking subway car where everyone was tense and unbalanced, trying to hang on and fight the swaying. Then I saw a man walking down the car, and his way of completely giving in to the lurching and swaying of the car was beautiful. He was really centered, flowing and yielding to the movements. Then when he sat down he collapsed in a heap, and I realized that he was dead drunk! Most of us waste so much energy fighting the forces around us when it is so easy to yield to them. You don't have to be drunk to let go and be more yielding.

Most dancers want to have a stereotyped body which is skin and bones with very long legs and arms. In fact, if you audition for certain ballet companies and your legs are not long enough, you cannot be accepted no matter how well you dance. So if you do not happen to be born with all that length you can become anxiety-stricken. You might say, "Maybe if I stretch my arms hard enough they will be a little bit longer." If you do this rigid stretching, your arm may measure a little longer but the movement dies and the gesture *looks* short. If you relax and just think of the feeling of the extension of the relaxed arm, it *appears* longer even though it is physically the same length. You do not measure human feeling by the length of the body, but by how it moves. If you give in to the feeling of your body, it extends for you, it curves.

Now let's try another variation of t'ui sho called "sticking-on," with some help from canned music. This tape sounds just like a bunch of birds that got trapped inside a room. It's a very strange sound; you know very clearly they are not out in nature. So when we do t'ai chi in this room, we are really in the same position as the birds.

Now, Arlene, you stick on to me—just follow me completely without any reservations. Stick with me, and don't lose me. A lot of things may happen to our two bodies if we allow them. All of you pair up and do this now. Let the sounds of the birds trigger your movement. Try anything, all directions and curves. See if the two of you can extend your flow into other bodies and connect with them so we can do chain movements. Stick on to someone else for a while, and then let go and find another person. When you play with exercises like this, and the feeling takes over, you feel every part of you is connected and alive. It's all coordinated some way, if you allow the movement to carry you. But the minute you begin to think, you're stuck.

Now I want to show you a different kind of t'ui sho, in which your hands move in a vertical circle. Begin by standing in a circle and use the center of the circle as your partner. Put your right foot forward and bring your right hand up to about chest level. Take three slow steps forward, and with your right hand make a complete vertical circle like a wheel rolling away from you. Then turn your arm toward you and let it circle back as the wheel is rolling back toward you. Imagine that you are a very playful elephant reaching out with your trunk to get a peanut, and then bringing it back to eat. It's a reaching out, gathering, and returning. You have the flexibility of the elephant's trunk instead of an arm with joints and angular movement. As you reach out, your whole arm faces outward as if saying, "Go away." As you gather in, your arm faces inward as if beckoning, "Come here."

Now choose a partner and do this with your hands together. As one of you moves forward in the yang part, the other moves backward in the yin part. As you do this, say "Go away" with your hand as you move forward, and "Come here" as you move backward. Let your whole body feel this circle and become part of this circular movement that connects you.

Play with each other's wrists as you wrap your hands around each other. The forward, aggressive move loops back into a retreating, receptive move. As you respond to your partner's advance, you move back, curving your hand towards yourself, gathering and receiving the energy coming to you.

When I work with some of you, I can sense your wrist pushing against me, meeting my contrasting energy. This makes it difficult for me to begin, because I have to try to match your leaning force, which is often too strong and unnecessarily tense. I have to fight you. When the forces become neutral, then it is possible for me to move with you. Then you are learning to listen with your body and match my energy accordingly. The tighter you try to hang on, the more you keep slipping off. Don't think of the contact as a tightly welded spot, and also don't melt into each other like Siamese twins. Just relax your wrist and elbow, feeling the contact and flowing with it. Feel it connect from the wrist, through the arm, spine, hip, legs, and down into your base. You can begin to realize your movement harmony within your body and with other bodies. You become aware of the connective, sequential flow. As you practice and become more sensitive; you will not be so self-conscious about the obvious parts of your physical self—arms, legs, etc. Your total sense of your physical-mental self will develop and become instinctively aware. You can't get this feeling by constantly checking on details intellectually; just allow the body to carry the mind into the unification of that all-of-you coming together.

As you continue to do this t'ui sho, I want to reflect on some of the things we have done. The other night in the folk-dancing session we really enjoyed ourselves and had a wonderful time. In the beginning you may find the structure of folk-dancing confining. You don't know the steps at all, so your first anxiety is to learn the step by watching the leader and then trying to match positions and you get all uptight. I went around the circle and took your hands, hoping to make your realize we were doing t'ui sho as we were doing the grapevine step. If your hand is not relaxed, how can you possibly follow the person next to you either to the right or to the left? You can slip into the rhythm of the steps of the folk-dancing by following and allowing the movement to carry you. Then you don't have to struggle to learn it intellectually.

We did mostly Greek and Israeli dancing with a marvelous sense of earthiness and vigor. In this kind of dancing there is usually singing along with the spirit of the motion. If you allow the singing and the sense of the movement to flow through you without worrying, then the dancing will come to you. Also in each folk dance the movement pattern repeats several times, so that by the end you can learn the dance by just doing it. The t'ui sho we're practicing now is so repetitious you may ask, "Do I get anywhere?" You don't get anywhere, and if you are really involved in it, you don't ask such questions.

It's very important to not make t'ai chi too solemn.

You often see people practicing t'ai chi quite concentrated. There is a hush and everything stands still, *except* the moving body. Don't make it an antiseptic, sacred, exotic, oriental thing. T'ai chi can be just as much fun as folk-dancing. You should sing inside. T'ai chi is a dance in its most pure form, suspended and crystallized. It is an unlimited resource. You can *see* it and *feel* it and *hear* it. Is your body moving like the sound of the ocean? Like the crackling of the fire log? The wind? The space between leaves on a tree? Or are you moving like arranged pieces of furniture, very consciously put-together?

When we go away from the man-made structure of the city and look at nature, we sense a special feeling of release and awe about the natural arrangements of things. We look at the mountain top and say, "Wow, it's beautiful!" Very few of us have the audacity to say, "Oh, that's not balanced. According to what I learned in art appreciation class, that particular hill is slightly lopsided. We must add a mound of rock over there to balance it." "That tree is too short, it's not balanced with the other tree there, and this brook is meandering the wrong way according to my idea of design. We must switch it around." The only time this attitude works at all is when you try to imitate nature, for instance to make a garden in your own back yard.

In Chinese gardening, the designer tries to allow nature to flow. The gardener doesn't say, "I am so artistic, that's why I can make something beautiful." Instead he says, "If I allow myself to flow as an instrument of nature, then my doing will also be a thing of nature. I will mold according to nature's demands." Then whatever he has designed and arranged will be a result of his meditation with nature.

Likewise in t'ai chi the nature of your body is master. You don't say, "Now, muscle in the arm, do this; bone in the leg, do that." If you do, you will get hopelessly confused when the movement becomes more complex. You have to allow the collection and the expansion of your center to work for you. Your body will become a very coordinated, unified orches-

tral composition. Allow the sound to take over. Don't
be the conductor all the time. You raise your baton
once to begin and that's enough. Eventually even the
first movement of the baton will be spontaneous.

It's like the story of the centipede who was walking along fine until someone asked him how he managed all those legs. If he starts thinking about each
individual leg, then his brain cannot possibly co-
ordinate it all. All the energy, all the musculature
within all those many legs must unite and collect into
one simple crystallized action. Just as the many legs of
the centipede must unite into one coordinated action,
all possibilities of the t'ai chi movement must settle
into one clear beginning.

Mind and body are one. We must learn to move
our body and mind together again. Bodymind, mind
underneath body, body floating over mind, mind go
around body, bodymind emerging and coming around
in a big round sphere—moving, fusing. When we
worry about each detail, we stop. Detail by itself only
bogs us down, but the whole sense of one/together
works. Then there's a whole happiness of releasing
and giving, and dance happens. Dancing is the energy
gathering in, flowing out. There's a wonder, and a
sense of discovery.

I'm still a fairly new father and I find great joy
in watching my daughter. She dances with me a lot,
and she always has a new approach to familiar things.
When she wakes up in the morning we always share
a special time together. We have our little routine.
She has her juice and a bowl of cereal. It seems that
each morning there is a different way of asking for
the juice, drinking the juice and eating the cereal,
looking out at the flowers, saying the same words,
repeating what she has discovered about the birds
or the squirrels or the flowers.

Being close to a child helps us to rediscover childlikeness in ourselves. A child *is* spontaneous: he
doesn't *try* to be. Spontaneity *comes*—it just flows,
like rain. Thunder comes, trees grow, flowers open.
You don't force a flower to open; it opens by itself.

Your self does, too. Let your self be self. Not in an egotistic sense but just allowing that manifestation to happen, so that each one of us moves and dances out of our own accord.

T'ai chi moves from stillness, like the opening and closing of a flower. Close your hand into a fist and look at it. Now open it up slowly, and see the fingers open. See the space between your fingers and feel the sensitive flow and the warmth inside of your palm. Close that space in, and then open out. T'ai chi is that in-and-out alternation—the expansion/contraction interchange—the process of allowing these seemingly two extreme feelings to coexist and merge. If you explore the middle range of your grasp, you will feel less pulled apart by the two extremes. The extremes and the range in between are all the possibilities of life. Sometimes we feel like a tight fist; other times we feel ourselves extending too far, and getting further and further away. But it's that feeling of mid-range process that keeps us in balance.

Now raise your arms in front of you and make a circle with your arms by touching the tips of your fingers together. Do you see the empty circle in front of you? This is also a part of your body. Look at the solid circle of your arms. But what about the space in between your arms? Do you negate that? Do you say that's not your body, that it has nothing to do with you? It has everything to do with you. You are enclosing it; it becomes you.

The space between your legs also gives you balance in the t'ai chi base. If you concentrate on the yin space, you relieve your anxiety and the tension in your legs. Then the muscles will relax. Otherwise your thighs may get very tight and sore.

Use your hands to lightly touch all around the inside and outside of your thighs and legs down to your knees, so you can feel the sensitivity of your skin. It's that sensitivity to the space that gives your base a lift and allows you to move without tensing.

Now lift one leg up in front of you until your thigh is horizontal, with your lower leg relaxed and dangling. Use your hands underneath your thigh to support your leg so you don't need to use any lifting muscles in your leg. Get that feeling of being supported. Then try the other side. Now lift your leg without using your hands, and see if you can keep the same feeling of being supported, using the space beneath your leg.

This balance on one leg looks like a motif called the Golden Rooster. Lift your right leg in front of you, relaxed, with knee bent until your thigh is horizontal. The right arm rises at the same time, as if the arm is pulling the leg up with invisible strings. Then the elbow drops slightly and the supporting knee softens as you settle into your tant'ien. Now bring your right arm and leg down and repeat the same movement on the other side. Breathe in as your leg rises so you can ride on top of the breath. You don't pick up your leg; you push away from the standing leg, and ride on the space underneath the lifting leg. Bounce on that leg. Let the spring-action reverberate like an echo as the leg rests.

With each lift, each transformation of your shape, think of the movement in the space around you. As you lift up, think of your arm and leg resting on the space underneath. Balance must be that mutual cooperation of yin space and yang space. This will relieve you of the anxiety of trying to reach a particular position and then having to hold it. Imagine that the space beneath you pushes you up as you move. As you do this, keep feeling the energy going upwards, between the legs, lifting to the center. Each rebound and kneebend should have that feeling of uplift. Otherwise you feel squat, and pretty soon you will be walking like a duck.

Find the center line at the top of your head, and pull the hair up with one hand, to remind yourself that your torso is going upward as you move. Now dig in and go down even further, so that you can rebound even higher. Underneath your torso two legs are bouncing up. You have to go down in order to come up again. That two-way stretch feeling should be there, with the energy from below and the energy from above meeting and returning. You send energy out and bring it back. You don't lose it: It always curves from infinity back to you. Let the energy move in your spine—it goes up and curves outward and downward and then back upward as you take it from the earth.

In the *Tao te Ching* there's one chapter saying that when you reach, you go farther away; and when you go farther, you curve; when you curve farther, you return; and finally you come back to yourself. Here you can discover this in your movement. If you let energy flow, the body will do whatever it must to adjust to it. When one energy cannot go any farther, then you curve, revolve, return, continue to shift weight to reach balance as you become centered again. T'ai chi helps us to transcend the physical limitation of what we are: the limitation of what you think you can do with that body of yours. We have only so much body, but it's as *if* the body is limitless when we understand that curve of movement.

Next I would like to do a simple motif called the Five Elements. The five elements are fire, water, wood, metal, and earth. This is an important motif to give you a sense of orientation in the four directions. Most Chinese masters insist that you begin by facing north. But here, I like to begin facing the ocean which is really the west. Why does it have to be north? If you're in a room in which the only pleasant corner is the southwest, why not face that?

Begin by stepping forward on your right foot as you push out with the same movement we used in the an. This is the fire or energy step, in which you can imagine that fire shoots out of your palms.

The natural return from fire is, of course, the water step. As you pull the energy back toward you and receive it, you shift your weight back onto your left foot. Then you turn to your left and let your palms rotate out and curve out, and back around to your right. This wide sweeping circular movement out and to the right is the element of wood or growth.

You continue turning to the right until you can't turn any more without moving your feet. This extreme twisting and turning is the metal element. To resolve it, you bring your left leg around under you and return to the fifth element, earth, the center. You gather in the energy and lift it up and settle it into your belly. This is the same movement as the Embrace Tiger, Return to Mountain sequence we did earlier.

Now you find that your direction has turned a quarter-turn to your right. After you repeat this four times you return to face in the same direction you originally started.

The simple lession of the Five Elements sequence in the creativity of tao is explained this way: The fire is the ch'i, the energy, the yang coming out of you. This then has to be quickly received and balanced by the water which is the receptive, giving, yin step. When yin and yang unite, the birth of a new open movement becomes wood—an expression of natural life and growth. Then you briefly pass through the metal curve and resolve back into earth. It's very possible for the metal to be destructive and hard. Like the sword, it is deadly when used wrong, so you immediately move this destructive energy down into the earth.

Some of you need more of a sense of an all-around base. The minute you feel "front leg" and "back leg," you are in trouble. The front and back leg must become one leg in the middle. It's your root. Imagine that your legs are like a tree trunk with strong roots going out into the ground in all directions. Think of *one*, instead of two separate supports.

In our culture neither men nor women are supposed to sit with their legs open. So we usually sit with legs crossed or close together. The sense of space between your legs becomes less and less, and you lose the awareness of that circular support under you. We joke about the cowboy who walks along as if the horse is still there. But what we see in his body is what we should feel in our own. In the Orient, men used to wear very bulky pantaloons. The heavy fabric between their legs must have reminded them of that space in the middle.

Even as you step forward, think of *oneness,* so the leg will be in the middle. Think of one, think of the circle; don't let it become two. The minute you separate them, you have to rely on one leg and drag the other around. Begin with your legs parallel. Don't turn your legs out too wide, because this presents two different directions.

When you practice the Five Elements sequence, wait until you feel the fire coming out of your palms before you step forward. Let the energy flow. Otherwise your ch'i will get stuck in your hands and your body will feel congested. After you have done the pattern four times in one direction and have made a complete revolution, then do it in the other direction with the other leg forward. Don't get confused by doing it in the other direction. Just remember to turn toward the open side, the natural side. This is important: This is the organic part of t'ai chi which you have to experience. Otherwise you will always do this step awkwardly, trying to remember what somebody said, instead of following the flow of the movement. If you are thinking and remembering, then you lose the awareness of your body and your surroundings.

As you move you can follow the whole unity of your right arm and your left arm, your neck and your shoulder, your right knee and your left hip, your right toe and your left heel. All the intricate parts of you play the orchestra of your movement. They are waiting for you to let go, so they can come together. Most of the time we block them off, we stop them from moving together according to their own rapport.

As you open up to your own body, you also open up to the world around you. Then you find yourself moving and being content to let this movement carry you without your interference.

Usually when I walk in the moonlight I see my shadow on one side or the other. But last night there was no shadow because the moon was directly over my head. "High moon." You can feel the heat of the sun and you can get a tan. No one I know can feel the moonlight or get a moon-tan. As I looked around, the moon was directly over my head, completely centered. It became me and all the moonlight in me and around me, invisible. Often I only appreciate moonlight by seeing the moon itself, instead of forgetting the moon and experiencing the moonlight around me, all over. It's a good image for what you experience when you begin to get settled and into the sense of being centered and suspended right in the middle. The moonlight comes from above, from below, from all over. You don't have to put your mind on an image outside, like watching a master or thinking about what to do. That's like looking at the moon all the time, having to have the moon there to tell you it's moonlight instead of just experiencing it.

Calligraphy

In this session I will illustrate t'ai chi through the medium of calligraphy, using brush and ink. First I will show you, and then we'll all work together. The preparation of the ink is painstaking, and serves as a centering process. You grind the inkstick on the stone in a circular motion. It's like being a potter, kicking the wheel and centering the clay. Usually I have a special place where I do calligraphy. I make an environment for myself where I can take my time to do this. It's much better to enjoy this grinding process than to just get a bottle of ink. Once in a while I may yield to the quickness of prepared ink when we do a group calligraphy session. When we roll the newsprint out and begin writing without stopping, we don't have time to work on getting more ink. But if you do it alone for yourself, it's a very important process. There is no need to rush.

I usually incorporate calligraphy in my t'ai chi sessions because it's another expression of the same discipline, another way of showing what we do in body movement. For instance, when we do the t'ui sho your hands move in a circle, and your whole body moves in relation to that circular movement. When I prepare the ink by this circular grinding, I'm going through the same circular process in my whole body.

The ink is ready now. I hold the brush with the t'ai chi fist—the empty open fist that is neither tense nor limp. The arm holding the brush is a resting arm, not a holding, rigid arm. As I dip the brush into the ink, all the hairs have to be smoothed to form a tip. This is as if a million different thoughts collect to one thin center point. The smoothing of the brush on the stone is another centering process.

When your brush is ready, you hold it in front of you vertically over the paper. The stem of the brush corresponds with your own spine. It's straight and hollow and flexible, and it is the center of movement. This is the beginning, and your awareness is right there at the center. In front of you is a piece of white paper. Nothing is on it. You meditate on it. If you were living in old China you would wear a gown with long, wide sleeves which would smear the ink on the paper. To prevent this, you hold both sleeves with the other hand, forming a circle with your arms. Now you approach the paper in the center. The usual sequence of strokes in Chinese calligraphy starts from left to right, and flows down and finishes at the lower right. Essentially it's a moving circle within a square design.

Watch the sequence of the strokes as this character (1.) develops. I begin with the first stroke at the top of the page. I sink the brush in and then immediately pick it up, forming a dot with a tail (2.). The next stroke begins slightly left of center and moves to center and then straight down to the bottom, finishing with an upward tail to the left (3.). This second stroke divides the space in half, establishing the spine of the character. The next four strokes balance and strengthen the character like the four limbs of the body. The third stroke goes from left to center and the fourth stroke moves down and left (4.). The fifth and sixth strokes mirror the previous two on the other side of the center line (5.).

The first stroke means oneness or centering. The rest of the character means water. The whole character means forever flowing constancy: The oneness in the nature of the movement of water.

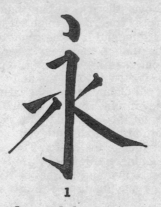

1

Notice the flow and the connection as one stroke leads into another. When you finish the last stroke, you keep the movement going, even after the brush leaves the paper. The energy of the brush stroke should go out to infinity, and then curve back. The curving transition in going from one stroke to another is parallel to the practice of t'ai chi movement. Beginners write each stroke separately, like a child. Because each stroke starts separately, with a different reference point, the character gets all lopsided. If you concentrate on the center as you write, using the t'ai chi feeling, each stroke is oriented toward that same point. The character will look centered and unified when you finish. I'm using the calligraphy discipline to illustrate this centering process. You can imagine your spine and body as the brush, and imagine your feet as the tip of the brush. You are doing your t'ai chi on the paper—or doing calligraphy on the ground. It's the same thing, and it's a part of you if you practice according to that discipline.

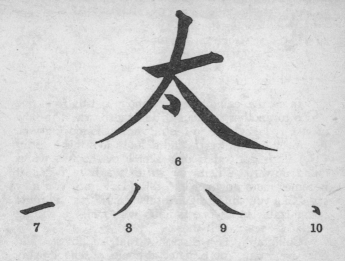

6

7   8   9   10

One of the most direct ways to show this parallel between t'ai chi and calligraphy is to ask you to superimpose your own body onto the Chinese character for t'ai (6.). Stretch your arms out to both sides with a horizontal undulation. This is the first stroke, a left-to-right horizontal line (7.). Then connect and slide the energy above your head down through your center spine and down through your left leg. This is stroke two (8.). Now move energy from your tant'ien downward and outward through the other leg. This is stroke three (9.), balancing the second stroke. The final stroke gathers up all the energy together in a concentrated dot in the center (10.). Use your right hand to pull all this energy together in a vigorous snatching motion right in your tant'ien.

When you write calligraphy, you should have a gliding smoothness, like the evenness of the t'ai chi circle. The brush stroke should have the same sensitive contact with the paper that you feel between your feet and the ground in t'ai chi. Beginners usually write with too much pressure in the tip of the brush and squash it.

11   12   13

In cursive calligraphy you move swiftly from one stroke to another without lifting the brush. The flow of energy takes over so the movement is moving you. For instance, the word "flight" looks like this in print (11.). It is derived from a sketch of the two wings going upward. When you write it a little faster, it becomes more flowing, like this (12.) until you may say, "Can you still recognize this (13.)?" It's still quite recognizable to anyone familiar with Chinese writing —the essence is still there.

Calligraphy is a discipline that a Chinese child does every day. You practice at home, at school, many hours each day until you get it. Both my parents are very fine calligraphers. I had the good fortune to enjoy all this practicing because of their inspiration and encouragement. Practicing the calligraphy technique gives me a wonderful sense of t'ai chi essence. Because you can see what you are writing, you can actually see this flow clearly. Sometimes when I teach calligraphy I will hold your hands as if you are a young child and just ask you to move with me. This is similar to the teaching of Balinese dancing. The teacher wraps around you from the back and you move together. All you have to do is just relax and absorb the movement from the teacher. But as I move your hand, often it will resist, so the character becomes very lopsided. If I ask you to use your left hand, the hand most of you do not use for writing, it usually doesn't have as much resistance. It follows me more easily, and the character comes out more balanced.

In calligraphy the brush becomes an extension of myself and the t'ai chi movement. My sword practice is based on the same principle. The sword also follows the curve and structure of t'ai chi movement as it slashes and cuts. I practice t'ai chi and then extend that into a weapon, like the sword, and play with its hardness and destructiveness. The sword is very yang, so I have to work the yin into it and find balance.

The sword practice also helps me to understand the difference between fulfillment and achievement; the difference between simply doing something well, and doing it *for* other people, or for me. Usually I resist practicing in a public place because people usually gather to watch. It's flashy and impressive to them, so they make me into a performer. But alone, I enjoy it simply because it feels good to manipulate and weave the weapon around. The sword that I've been using is an imitation of an old ritual sword, the taoist seven-starred sword. In the old days it was used for rituals having to do with changes in natural phenomena, like stars and planets. The seven stars on the blade represent the seven stars of the big dipper. It's a straight sword with two edges and is practiced as a solo weapon. It's quite different from the Japanese kendo sword which has a slight curve and only one edge.

The tip of the sword is called the mouth, and the edges are the teeth. The movement of the sword is the wind—it flows and curves like the wind. I use these images as I practice; they help me to feel the sword as a part of me that serves me. As I move through the form I become the sword and *we* become the movement.

The most important part of the practice is the beginning. I simply carry the sword in its sheath and walk slowly, sensing everything around me. When I feel energy gathering, I open up and draw the sword. I let it move with the energy until it settles, and then let the sword return to the sheath. The whole form is simply the drawing and returning of the sword. But *when* and *how* you draw it and return it is the meditation. There's another form practiced kneeling in which you wait alertly, yet relaxed, until the moment comes, and then you draw and rise to one of the eight directions.

The sword is held with the empty fist and relaxed wrist, just as the brush is held in calligraphy. One exercise is to revolve the sword in continuous vertical circles, rotating at the wrist. In order to continue the circle smoothly you cannot hold the handle tightly. Your hand is so relaxed that each time the sword comes around you let it go and catch it again just before it begins to slip. By holding it lightly you make this hard, destructive weapon soft and yielding. Perhaps there are a lot of hard edges of *you*, too, that need to be smoothed and curved as you work. The sword practice can help you to learn how to allow that swordlike part of you to come out in the open, so you can balance the yang with the yin. This sword is you, just as the brush is you when you write calligraphy.

Calligraphy is also an extension, another application of your t'ai chi practice. If some of you like to paint or already have a flair for using the brush, then this movement of the brush can be incorporated into your t'ai chi practice right away. Identify the t'ai chi feeling and bring it into whatever you are already doing. If you are a potter, then go back and center your clay with t'ai chi. If you are an architect, think and feel structure differently.

In a workshop with Alan Watts several years ago, the group decided that he and I should have a dialogue with calligraphy. We used the text of *Tao te Ching* as a structure to begin. We wrote very large on long rolls of newsprint in a big room. Our conversation became more heated as we began responding to each other faster and faster. We wrote cursively, and Alan's cursive became more improvisational. Suddenly neither of us knew what we were writing about. We were not concerned with the content; we were just flowing with the curving movement of the brush strokes.

As we kept rolling out the paper and writing, we heard a drum-beat begin: da, dada, da, da dum, dum —somebody was in the corner playing, and soon the group was dancing alongside the long strips of paper.

As the dancing became more energetic, feet began to tear the paper. Pretty soon torn paper was everywhere and the whole place was a whirlwind of energy and activity. Following a flying, looping curve of paper I danced over to the drummer to tell him how beautiful his playing was. And he shouted, "Oh, I got you, man. I feel it, I feel it."—and I realized that he was blind. He was just sitting there sensing our cursive conversation. I think the energy of the whole group transmitted that beautiful thing that was happening. This is what we want: the energy happening, and the t'ai chi emerging out of it.

Now you can all experience doing calligraphy. There are enough ink stones and blocks and brushes for all of you, so begin by making the ink. Hold the ink block upright and move it in an easy circular motion on the wet stone. It's best if you all stand up to do this, so your whole body can get into the motion. Remember what I said about the importance of making your own ink, as a centering and collecting process. Don't lose this opportunity to quiet yourself, or you will approach the calligraphy feeling scattered and unready.

This preparation slows you down, so you can see where the ink comes from, smell its fragrance and feel its blackness and thickness. Buying it in a bottle may be quicker but it's a little like seeing only frozen orange juice and thinking all oranges come in cans. A friend of mine went to Santa Barbara to visit someone. He looked out the living-room window at an orange grove and said, "My God! Oranges grow on trees!" He knows it very well, but still it's a revelation. Often we forget. The real miracle is the orange, not the instant can. So take some time with your ink and enjoy the process. Use it as a way of focusing your scattered energies.

Right now all of you surrounding me, with the rain falling outside, the soft light coming through the window, all provide an environment for us. We are slowing down, feeling comfortable as we prepare the ink.

Now hold your brush between the thumb and the index and middle fingers. Use the ring finger as a brace below the thumb, to help keep the brush upright. Now roll the spine of the brush around within your fingers. In t'ai chi, your own spine should feel as if it's being manipulated by the space around you in the same way that the brush is giving in to the fingers. The only way you will be able to move correctly is if you allow that outside energy to move you.

Right now we are standing in a circle. You are part of the circle, a part of all of us. You are also a part of the space between us, and a part of the rain, the soft light, the moisture in the air, everything here. You are moving inside of it. You're not outside looking in: you are within this wholeness.

You use the empty fist to hold the brush. Let your hand relax; let the brush float inside of your fingers. Don't clench your hand or this tension will spread throughout your body and your energy will get lost and congested.

Now draw the brush outward across the ink stone. Rotate the brush so all the hairs are drawn to make a tip that is as centered as possible. It's a nice easy stroke—like brushing someone's hair. This process of gathering a thousand hairs to one point is another way of gathering all your thoughts and scattered energy to one point of focus.

The brush should be full of ink, but don't saturate it until it drips down. When the brush is prepared, hold it in front of you, waiting for the movement to begin. There is a very important symbolism in the bamboo spine of the brush—it is round and its inside is hollow. It's not stuffed with things to make you feel heavy. It's air, it's flowing space, it's emptiness. There is also space between the inside of your hand and the contact with the brush—the empty fist. The five fingers come together in coordination, each one helping the others, while the empty space holds the centered energy. If you worry and think only about how to move your fingers, you will get stuck. Relax and let yourself rest into the unknown, the emptiness that lets the energy through.

Now draw an empty circle in space. This is the horizontal t'ui sho circle that we were doing. Now, reverse it and make a loop, an S-shape, an 8-shape, an infinity shape. See if you can continue the loop easily and still maintain that same sense of flow. And then get a little closer to the surface of the paper. Don't touch the paper yet, but just enjoy looking at its nice blankness.

The paper is still completely open and free. This is a good time to think of the distinction between a solid line and a suggested line. Which is more real? When I make a broken stroke, as in painting bamboo, the empty spaces between become very suggestive of something solid, like the joints of the bamboo. We describe this technique as "brush absent, idea present." We allow the white parts of the paper to suggest sky, snow, water or mist by painting dark areas of earth, mountain and trees. This way of utilizing the original whiteness of the paper corresponds to t'ai chi practice, in which we allow the moving empty space to complement the solid body—the yin and yang.

When the time comes to make the first stroke on the paper, let all your speculation about the outcome go—"Will it be good or bad?" "Will I want to frame it or burn it?" Just approach the paper empty, without prejudice. Let the first movement take over, like that first movement of t'ai chi ch'uan. Begin by making loops on the paper. Sense the connection between the brush and the paper without squashing the space in between.

Is it a nice, flowing, brushing feeling? Or are you dragging with a lot of friction between the tip of the brush and the paper? Allow your strokes to move off the paper and away from it. Don't let the edge of the paper confine you. The line doesn't have to stay within it. If you believe the suggested, empty line exists, you can fly right off the edge of the paper and come back onto it without feeling that the line has been interrupted. Try not to stand outside yourself and appreciate or depreciate what you have done. Don't try to make anything specific—moons or waterways or birds or smoke. If the lines remind you of something, fine. Let it remind you, and then let it go. If you happen to run into your neighbor's paper, fine—pick up his or her flow. By now you have many, many layers of lines and feelings and extensions on the paper. Look inside these layers of the lines you have made and trace their continuity. As you keep flowing over the paper, try not to let the clutter interfere with your energy flow, the smooth continuous path of the line.

When you feel your brush point is getting dry and off-center, go back to your ink stone and smooth it gently back again. At the same time, collect and center yourself until you are ready to begin. When you feel you need a clean sheet of paper, get it and begin again. I will move around and work with each of you. Let me support your hand once in a while, and try not to fight me. Relax into my movement with you. Try using your other hand as a support to the brush hand.

Keep your spine straight and free to move the brush, instead of tilting and turning the brush in your hand. Certain adjustments in your spine are necessary for different movements, but basically it must be centered with the brush upright.

Now you have done enough exploration; let me offer you some form, some discipline. Get a clean sheet of paper and find the center point of it. Draw the biggest circle you can around this center. Now divide the circle with an s-shaped line, forming a figure-eight. Now make variations of this double loop within the circle. Stand freely and let your body move with the curves. You are practically doing t'ui sho with your brush strokes. Continue to make loops on the paper, and fill up the whole space within the circle.

Now stand back, and look beyond the clutter of all those strokes. Transcend that mess of lines and retrace the process of what you have done, step by step

—back into the original yin/yang form you've made.
... back into the circle ... back into the empty page.
Keep all that feeling. Now, with one long breath, use
a continuous stroke to fill in all that space, until you
complete it with one last sweep off the paper.

14   15

I want to share this character with you now,
"Wind" (14.). It's a one-stroke word in cursive, one
of the fastest, easiest words to write. You can feel the
energy and follow it all the way through. When you
write wind in regular strokes, it breaks down into nine
strokes and looks like this (15.). But in cursive it
doesn't finish; it keeps looping around and then flies
off the paper.

I'll come around and make this character for each
of you. See if you can find your own sense of flow by
doing it yourself. I can see that the wind varies for all
of you—we have here a hurricane, a tornado, a gentle
breeze. This is a clear, fast, one-stroke, one-breath
expression that slides out of you into your brush. I
think when you play with this, the important thing is
to get that momentum going. See if you can stay
centered, and let the character come out in one breath
and finish without any stopping in the middle.

16

If you're ambitious, you can write this word,
"flight" (16.). Do you recognize the wind under-

neath? Flight is "riding on the wind." Move your brush through the empty space first without actually making the stroke for a few times, and see if you can follow the flow of the character. Ah! Someone just made a backwards flight. It's beautiful. It's backwards, but it's balanced in the t'ai chi circle.

山   馬   牜   川
17   18   19   20

There are two main kinds of characters, pictograms and ideograms. When you look at a pictogram, you can see a sketch or picture of what it represents. Mountain (17.) is a picture word. It's one big peak with a smaller one on each side. The character for horse (18.) is a sketch of the horse's neck and mane (19.) with the back and tail and four legs (20.).

For more abstract concepts, you have to create an ideogram—some way of representing a thought. Through the years characters were combined, with pictograms and ideograms mixed together and modified. Some of the original meanings get lost, and sometimes we have to find a new way of translating the characters. A character usually has a much richer meaning when you look deeply into the original meanings. English words also have more meaning when you look into their derivation from a word in Latin or some other archaic language.

This interpretation of Chinese characters can be very playful and creative. I don't let myself be bound by the historical meanings or the etymological derivations. I look at the strokes and the pictures they make, and interpret them through the feelings I get from each one. In China a very popular way of fortune-telling is called "taking words apart." There is someone who does this on nearly every busy streetcorner. If I want to ask him about my daughter's future, he might use her name or her birth date and take these characters apart. It's a little like numerology or reading tea leaves.

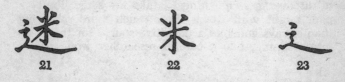

21 22 23

Some of you have been asking what your names mean in Chinese. We have only one-syllable words in Chinese, so we must find separate words for each of the syllables in your name. For instance, Michelle; the first word might be mi (21.), which means a sense of searching. The top of the character actually means rice, but it also looks like a symbol for the eight directions (22.). We can interpret it either as being centered where the eight directions converge, or as being lost with all the lines dispersing. The bottom part of the character (23.) is derived from "foot" or "path." It has gradually changed to look like a waterway, a flowing downward stroke. Mi is a word we use in children's games like hide-and-seek. Children know very well they are not really lost when they pretend to be. It can also mean the universal game of hide-and-seek all men play with their gods.

24 25 26

The second syllable of Michelle is harder, because there is no "l" sound in Chinese. I would use two characters to approximate the sound of "chelle" (24.). The one on the left (25.) means "rain crystallizes," or "snow." The one on the right (26.) means "child." Together they mean "child of snow." My personal interpretation of the whole name Michelle is this: "Child of snow, play the game of being lost. In searching, don't get confused with too many choices of directions—simply ride over the way of the water."

When I interpret Chinese playfully, I never cease to discover new meanings. I take the same liberty a poet might with words. It is much more satisfying than always going to a definitive source for the absolute meaning, like a careful researcher would do.

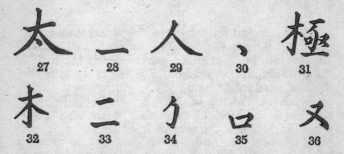

Now let's look at the two words t'ai chi. T'ai (27.) consists of four clear strokes. The first stroke is "one" (28.). The second and third strokes make "man" (29.). The fourth stroke, the dot, is "center" (30.). T'ai means "the centered man." The left side of the character chi (31.) is "wood" (32.), a tree with trunk and branches. On the right, the top and bottom lines (33.) symbolize heaven and earth. "Man" (34.) is in the middle, between heaven and earth. On one side of the man is "mouth" (35.), and on the other side is "hand" (36.). The character chi means the extremes, the poles, or man's eternal struggle between the larger universe of heaven and earth and his own internal essence of the uncarved block—his true self or basic nature. When we put t'ai and chi together, we reach a perfect balance.

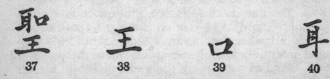

Another similar character (37.) is usually translated as sage, or wise man. The lower part (38.) means "king," a man centered between heaven and earth. Above are the characters for ear (39.) and mouth (40.). The wise man listens as he speaks—he takes in and gives out. A sage is a perceptive and quiet man.

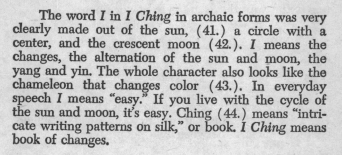

41   42   43   44

The word *I* in *I Ching* in archaic forms was very clearly made out of the sun, (41.) a circle with a center, and the crescent moon (42.). *I* means the changes, the alternation of the sun and moon, the yang and yin. The whole character also looks like the chameleon that changes color (43.). In everyday speech *I* means "easy." If you live with the cycle of the sun and moon, it's easy. Ching (44.) means "intricate writing patterns on silk," or book. *I Ching* means book of changes.

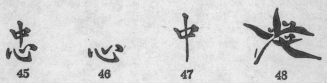

45   46   47   48

All parents in China pick nice names for their children. My name Chung (45.) means "centered-heart." The character for heart (46.) is placed centered at the base. Floating above it is an arrow hitting a bulls-eye (47.). Heart is a very beautiful character. It looks like a bowl, with energy flowing out of it, spilling over, like a fountain. These same strokes are used in Chinese painting for the stamens of an orchid (48.). So it's also like the heart of a flower, the center of its unfolding.

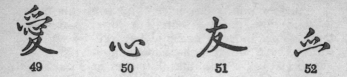

49   50   51   52

Heart also appears in the word commonly used for "love" (49.). Heart (50.) is in the middle. Below it is a character meaning friendship or relationship (51.). The top part (52.) doesn't have a fixed meaning, but it has the feeling of slow unfolding. If you put this all together, you get "the slow unfolding of heart relationship." When you love, you relate to others the way the heart of a flower opens.

53   54   55

A different character for "love" is (53.). This part (54.) is "man." This part is "two" (55.). The whole character means "between two people."

56   57

The Chinese characters with many strokes are much more difficult to write. Here is a word I use all the time, "dance" (56.). This is a fifteen-stroke word. The number of strokes can go as high as thirty-five. This word, "the transformation" (57.), has twenty-six strokes. All those twenty-six strokes must form a balanced, centered whole.

The meaning of another complex word, *yü* (58.) is "melancholy." Within this character there are many parts. This part (59.) is "wood" or "tree." One tree

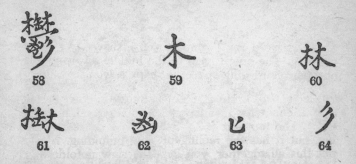

58   59   60

61   62   63   64

is fine; it's uncluttered. Two trees (60.) become "woods." With more than two trees—especially all growing in different ways—we have jungle and confusion (61.) Underneath the confused jungle, we see a lopsided rice field (62.). And below that is the character for "knife," upside down (63.) which looks like going into a corner. Fortunately the last part of the character (64.) consists of three parallel lines moving downward. These provide a balance to the confusion, and suggest that it is possible to flow out of it.

65   66   67

In speech we often precede *yü* with *yú*, which is also a troubled character, meaning "worry" (65.). The bottom part of yú is identical to the word "love." But on top is a single stroke meaning "one" (66.) and a character for "self" (67.). Instead of the spontaneous unfolding that is at the top of the character for "love," there is a man withdrawn into himself, not relating to others. A playful translation could be "man underneath the roof, crying over heart matters—should be friendship." This is definitely self-created worry.

68

The word for "woman" (68.) shows two arms cradling. The open space in the middle also suggests an open nourishing space, perhaps a womb.

男   田   力

69   **70**   **71**

The word for "man" (69.) also tells a story. The top part shows the square outlines of a divided rice field (70.). The bottom part (71.) means "strength." So "man" means "strength in the field."

性   十   生

72   **73**   **74**

There is no character in Chinese that is the exact equivalent of the English word for "sex," but there's one character that is used to translate everything sexual in western psychology books (72.). The left part of the character (73.) is derived from "heart," and the other part (74.) means "birth" or "human essence." In everyday Chinese, it really means "man's nature in the beginning."

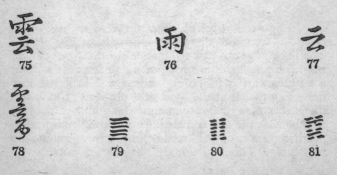

75   **76**   **77**

78   **79**   **80**   **81**

The character for sexual intercourse in Chinese is "cloud and rain." The character for cloud (75.) shows rain (76.) becoming vapor (77.). I'll write cloud and rain altogether in cursive (78.). It's really "rain/vapor/rain." Because there is cloud there is rain; because there is moisture in the air, there is cloud. It's the continuous changing cyclical transformation of rain to vapor to rain. In the interpretation of *I Ching*, the clouds are formed and rain falls as a result of the harmonious union of the yin and yang forces. The first two hexagrams Ch'ien (19.) and K'un (80.) transform into another hexagram K'an (81.) by mutual penetration. In the symbolic translation of K'an, the upper trigram is always referred to as cloud, and the lower one as rain, even though they are identical.

82   83   84   85

"Pregnancy" (82.) is also a nice character. It shows the beautiful curve of a pregnant woman's breast and belly (83.). Inside the belly where the baby would be is a small character (84.) that means "again" or "another." At the bottom is the character for "child" or "offspring" (85.).

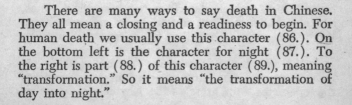

86   87   88   89

There are many ways to say death in Chinese. They all mean a closing and a readiness to begin. For human death we usually use this character (86.). On the bottom left is the character for night (87.). To the right is part (88.) of this character (89.), meaning "transformation." So it means "the transformation of day into night."

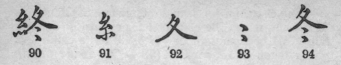

90   91   '92   93   94

Another character for death or ending is (90).
On the left side is the character for silk (91.). On the
right side is the character formed from "long night"
(92.) and "snow" (93.), meaning "winter" (94.). The
whole could be translated as "when winter comes and
the silkworm finishes spinning."

了

95

Here is another character for death (95.). It
simply shows that you have finished whatever you're
saying.

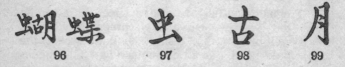

96   · 97   98   99

Butterfly is two characters (96.). The left part of
the first character shows an arrow and bulls-eye symbol (97.), and means "insect." The middle part means
"ancient" (98.). The last part is the "crescent moon"
(99.). So we have "the insect of the ancient moon."
The left part of the second character of butterfly is
the same as the first: "the insect." The right side
means "leaf," which describes the butterfly's wings,
and also has a sense of unfolding or metamorphosis.
When we put it all together we have something like
"a leaflike insect of an ancient moon."

If I add the character for "dream" (100.), we
have Chuang Tzu's "butterfly dream." On the top is
the character for "grass" (101.) which also means

100

101

102

103

"springing up" or "emerging." In the middle we have a horizontal eye (102.), which signifies that it is closed, sleeping. At the bottom is the character for "night" (103.). The dream.

Most Chinese teachers do not take words apart this way or explain much to you—at least not the ones I had in school. But if you are a person who likes to really understand, then one day during calligraphy session you discover, "Ohhhh! Woooo! That's what it means! Yes, it *is* dream!"

There's so much intrinsic wisdom in the Chinese language. Unfortunately most people stop at the obvious and allow the words to be abstract. Unless you submerge yourself in the character, and fully experience it, you only see a nice combination of meaningless strokes, and it loses its richness of meaning. It can be a storytelling picture, a feast of ideas, multidimensional. A brush stroke is only a stroke; the meaning and wisdom is between the lines.

I enjoy calligraphy very much because I keep discovering things. I like to have fun with it and let my intuition take over. I used to do calligraphy for one reason or another, but never for *myself*. I used to practice diligently for my father. I remember his coming to the study to watch us practice. He would circle the characters he liked with a special red ink brush. By the end of the week, we children would count the red circles. And if we had enough, he would take us to Sunday tea or some other treat.

I practiced hard for my teachers, too. They would hold and move our brush-hands, patiently helping us to find the balance of each character. Often we copied directly on top of pre-printed red characters. Other times, we wrote over a clearly drawn geometri-

104

105

cal design (104.) to help us develop symmetry and balance. For instance, the character "water" (105.) fits perfectly into this design. The first stroke down the middle falls on the vertical line and the four side strokes fall on the diagonals of the square.

After many years of practicing structurally like this, you begin to acquire your own sense of centering and balance. Eventually you find that the red character of the geometric design is unnecessary. Then you begin to write flowingly, connecting one stroke to another, condensing, simplifying, leaving one or two lines out, but carrying the energy through. You pause less and less, and finally you sweep through the whole character with one stroke, in one breath cycle, writing cursively. Notice how quickly you arrived at the cursiveness in your brushwork this afternoon. You were learning it the creative way. There was no need to go through the usual painstaking apprenticeship. Very few of you are concerned about becoming a great calligrapher in three hours. You have been enjoying the process, and you have had a taste of the creative essence.

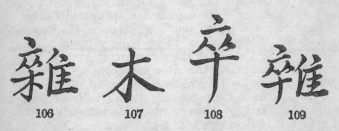

106   107   108   109

O.K., let's rinse our brushes, rinse the stones, and collect all the debris. Here is one of the characters

for debris (106.). Oh! that's interesting. I just discovered that this character for debris comes from a
battle scene. All these men—bodies of soldiers (107.)
in the woods (108.) together with the dead birds
(109.). Every character allows a particular interpretation at a particular time, because it's flexible. It's like
reading a hexagram: Depending upon when you do
it, and how perceptive you are at the moment, you
read it differently. But of course the underlying truth
will always remain.

Zen Ox Pictures

There are many versions of the ten zen ox pictures. I have given you two sets to pass around and look at.* I have deliberately mixed them up before giving them to you, because I want you to look at each one individually before seeing them in sequence. One version is in circles and the other version has a square outline. In most of the pictures you see a boy or young man. In some pictures you see him alone, and in some pictures you see him with an ox or a water buffalo. There is always some kind of nature around: trees and water, moon and stars. In each picture you see a particular relationship between the man and the ox.

In one version you see also the change in color of the ox. This series is also called "the whitening of the ox." The ox is all black in the first picture and gets whiter and brighter as you go through the ten pictures. The ox is a symbol of man's nature, and these pictures are a metaphor of man and his own nature. It's a way of presenting guidance regarding man's struggle with himself that is used in Zen Buddhism.

There are ten pictures, and when you think in circles, any one of them can be the beginning of the series. That's why I mixed them up when I gave them to you. I don't want you to worry about where you are in the sequence, especially when these zen pictures

---

* Please see the insert of this book for these pictures.

are used as a tool for a continual discipline of reflection. Let me put all the pictures in sequence now and I will go through them with you. I'll go first into the circle version.

The first picture (plate I) and the poetic text describes the boy searching for the ox. The poetry is an elaboration of the visual metaphor. We see the water rising, rapids, a waterfall, a whirlpool. We see the distant mountains and a falling star. We see flying clouds and endless path into distance. The boy is alone, searching in the wilderness, in the jungle or woods. He is lost. He has lost his ox. He is tired, confused, in despair. Perhaps he turns his head to hear the cicadas singing nearby.

In the second picture (plate II) the boy begins to acquire an attitude of looking towards one direction. He is finding some direction within his sense of his surroundings. The poetry commentary says that by the water, under the tree, he sees the tracks of the ox. The grass is very deep and smells very fragrant. When the spring wind blows, it almost smells like the flowers in his home garden. There are a lot of wild beasts running around, looking up, snorting, stamping the ground, but the boy doesn't sense them. We begin to realize that the animal and the man's heart are really one metaphor. But it is mostly hidden, only sometimes appearing—hide and seek.

In the third picture (plate III) he hears the nightingale, he follows the wave of the willow branches. The sun is very warm, the wind is very soft, the water is cool. Suddenly he sees the tail of the ox flapping. Now he sees the back of the ox. He sees a very strong body with big horns. The energy is very yang, very masculine. This is when he first discovers the ox; he begins to see traces of his own nature.

In the fourth picture (plate IV) the boy begins to encounter the ox. They move in a circle, looking at each other. The boy approaches the ox. But the animal's instinct, his unruly, ungoverned nature, is very difficult to tame. This is the beginning of catching and taming.

In picture five (plate V) the boy—perhaps myself

—and the ox become acquainted. Now the ox turns around and completes the circle with me. We talk and answer. We struggle. We go forward and we retreat together. Finally I put a rope through his nose; I tame the ox.

Number six (VI): I am riding the ox, returning home. In the evening mist I play the flute, I hear the echo in the valley singing back with me. My heart is calm. The ox and I are riding on the wind.

Number seven (VII): I have arrived home. The ox is not there. I've forgotten him. I kneel down, looking at the moon. I'm dreaming of far-away places, the edge of the heavens. I pick up the whip that I used to tame the ox. It's useless. I throw it away.

Number eight (VIII): The man and the ox both disappear. All is essence, all is greatness, all is emptiness. Heaven is very high. The earth is very wide. There are floating clouds, there is drifting snow. Wild fire, spring wind. Everything dissolves.

Number nine (IX): The return to the source. Wanting to retain the memory, already you are lost. It's better to have never left home. Not straining to see and listen, be like the blind and deaf. Do not interfere with nature. Quietly I watch the running water. The flower opens, the millions of colors appear and who knows why?

Number ten (X): Opening my heart, bare-chested, barefoot, I come to the busy corner, the downtown area, the open field. I have dust on my brow, but I have very broad eyes. I do not need the help from heaven. I point to the wintry branches, and flowers burst open.

That's one version of the ten pictures. This other version is more concentrated: It eliminates the first period of seeing the traces, following the traces and beginning to see the ox. The first picture (XI) begins immediately with encountering the ox, which is completely black in color. Over the ox is a black cloud. The text says: The ox is snorting, panting and very energetic. There is the yang, the masculinity, the strength of the ox. It is running, galloping over the hill, over the wild field, with the horns pointing straight up to the sky. He runs so far he has lost his way. Over his head at the entrance of the valley the clouds gather and become very dark, sweeping over very gentle, small fine grass. But the hooves of the ox do not know the nature of being gentle.

In the second picture (XII) the discipline begins. This is the beginning of the experience of being controlled. The essence of nature, of wildness, is struggling with the forces of discipline. The ox is wild and energetic, but the man insists on harmony. Finally, the boy passes the grass rope through the nose of the ox; the connection is made between the ox and the man.

Number three (XIII): The ox is following the rope, going with the man. Now the ox's head is white. He is going through water, over water, around the mountain paths: To the end of the world, to the edge of the sea he follows. Every day the man and the ox persevere and work very hard. The creative energy never stops.

Number four (XIV): The knowledge. The external learning becomes deeper, thicker. Seeing and listening become wider, vaster. The center of the heart seeks outwardness. Finally, the ox turns its head, looking at me. We look at each other; we have nothing to say. My enemy has become my friend. The animal nature has become tamed. But I am not confident. I cannot believe it. I continue to keep the rope in his nose, and I tie it to the willow tree. With confidence, while guarding the tree, I sing. I see the flower blossoms on the tree, but I do not dare to venture far away from the tree.

Number five (XV): Underneath the willow tree by the brook, next to the ancient mountains and the old rocks, I untie the rope. I welcome the wind. I feel the freedom, the spontaneity. I imitate the quality of the wind and water and the quietness and calmness of the mountain and the rock. Suddenly the evening mist becomes very cold. The green pastures seem to be behind me, far away. I find myself with the ox, returning home.

Number six (XVI): The ox is sitting very quietly; it seems old and settled. Now only its tail is still black. We turn our heads, looking at each other. Very happily I sing to myself and play my flute. The melody is very sweet, like the flow of water. Underneath the pine tree the air is calm, and I feel very peaceful, very contented. The flower of my heart opens out like the needles of the pine tree.

Number seven (XVII): The branches of the plum tree bend and move with the wind. The evening sun sinks into the green between the leaves. Water flows, I sit by the bank. Now the ox is all white. He drinks when thirsty, grazes when hungry. There is green grass, very deep, very dark. I do not know in my sleep how many birds have been singing, how many petals have fallen. How wide, how vast is the sky, and how enduring is the earth. Is it just a moment passing?

Number eight (XVIII): The ox has become completely transparent. The white cloud also has no shadow. I do not know which is the man, and which is his shadow. Man and ox, both quite happy to be. The moonlight casts white shadows, each without form. The stars and the moon are embracing, giving out the same light.

Number nine (XIX): The seven stars encircle the moon. The ox has disappeared, and only the man remains. I am my master. I am my king. I am like a small cloud drifting over the peaks of the mountain. I clap my hands, and the mountain answers. I sing joyously, and the moonlight echoes back my singing. But I am looking for the entrance of heaven, the gate of my home. The returning path is curving around.

Last picture (XX): Both the man and the ox are forgotten. There's no shadow, no trace of either. The moonlight is very empty, and very white. All the stars seem to fall and gather within the whiteness. The clouds gather, formless, shapeless. Ten thousand moving things. What is the meaning of all this? Contemplate the lilies, the green pastures, the scent, the quietness, and the swallow's flight. The butterfly and myself perhaps are one. Emptiness, void, emptiness. Fulfillment, fullness, happiness. What is the meaning of all this? The great tao. Ahhhh!

That's one of the many versions of the verbal text describing the true sense of the pictures. I translate it easily, unpurposefully, just looking at the Chinese characters, so I can relate for you exactly what the characters literally say in bits and pieces. These zen pictures have been used for students of life as a very basic way of learning and moving toward a state of what we call enlightenment or satori. Satori means a sudden enlightenment, which is usually not a lasting thing. Usually in the first picture you have a stage of being lost, searching. Then you see the traces of the ox. Then you encounter the ox and struggle to tame him and make friends with him. Finally you become one with the ox, and the ox and you both disappear. This sequence is based on the paradox of looking for your glasses when you're riding on it. It's like looking for your glasses when they're on your forehead.

The first version (I–X), the more common one, has one additional picture after the man and ox have both disappeared. The man is old now; he comes back to the world, entering the market place looking very jolly, bare-chested, carrying a gourd. You study zen to attain that emptiness in which all is fullness. After you attain that, what do you do? Return to the world and let the fullness of the world into your emptiness. The last picture shows the enlightened man quite simple—a very uncluttered man who has very little aura of being the "great man." He appears to be a beggar or a hermit—someone quite unimpressive in the everyday superficial sense of success. The gourd he carries is a symbol of emptiness. He has a bundle of goods that he gives away. His smile seems to say, "I know, but I don't know how to tell." The whole cycle begins again. There is a young man facing him, stooping down, just beginning his journey, his search. You can take this as a whole lifetime of searching.

You might say the first picture (I) is the time of a young man's life. I am searching now. I have a goal. I fight for it and finally I achieve it. Then I discover that the superficial achievement is not important. Therefore, I understand the essence of zen and arrive at enlightenment. I transcend that into the whole union between what is the physical external achievement, and what is really valuable out of myself.

Many people like to identify themselves with the zen ox pictures. "I am at this stage, I am at picture number four. This is the way I look at me now: The ox's head is white, the body is still black. This is the way I am with myself now. I am still leashing myself with a straw rope. Ah, wouldn't it be nice to be able to ride home on the ox's back, playing the flute?" It's fun to identify in this way. You can also use these pictures for short events and journeys that we encounter every day. *Within* each situation you may have this whole cycle. Events happen and yield to emptiness, and then you experience the emptiness. Soon it will gather dust. Later on it will be full of ~~~ and will look just like the ~~~ your body feels like the ~~~

Perhaps. If you practice t'ai chi or some other discipline, perhaps by evening you will have returned to the source. At night you may come out and laugh and dance like an idiot—like the bare-chested, barefoot man carrying an empty gourd. Idiot sounds so bad in English, but the zen idiot is different. There are many characters like this in Chinese literature. The zen idiot laughs at the moon and runs in the wind like a child.

The picture of the ox and man both gone is number eight (VIII). It could be number one. Sometimes you are lucky enough to begin this way. Most of us did begin this way when we were first born. Many people have encountered these pictures and the very beautiful poetry and ideas. But we may get bogged down and stuck with one particular description. All these different versions of saying what it is, really don't amount to anything special. It's just a description of the very natural flow of our human development.

I will just quickly summarize the themes of the pictures in the second (XI–XX), more concise, version: The ox is undisciplined. The beginning of harmony, beginning of taming. The turning around, the taming. Unfettered, no obstacle between. Then you follow the movement. Looking, reflecting, alone. Solitary moon, looking at the moon, reflecting the completeness and emptiness of the moon after the ox has disappeared. Both man and ox forgotten. Emptiness. A complete circle. Now the cycle begins all over again.

The other version (I–X) starts out a little earlier. It starts even before the undisciplined realization. You are in the middle of nowhere, unaware. You don't even have anything to discipline. You don't know how to discipline. But there is some sense of you, within the complex natural phenomena—the cloud, the mountain pass, the water, the trees, the wind. Then you see the traces, your path, your direction. You find your goal, your master, your guru. Then you wrestle with it. You tame, you follow, then you ride home with it. Riding on a water buffalo is a very common metaphor. In China you often see a small boy riding home on a water buffalo, playing his bamboo flute. Next you and the ox are one, so the ox has no need to be in the picture. You are alone. This aloneness is very different from the first picture when you are lost and you haven't yet found anything of you. Now you have the sense of the ox within you. Then you are both forgotten, returning to the purity of emptiness.

This comes from the Buddhist idea that all our sense of existence is mostly illusion. This world of illusion bursts, like a bubble. But where does this bubble burst into? Back to nature, back to your own roots; you return to the source. The very last picture (X) is more of a moral guidance. Now that you've attained enlightenment, what's next? Do you just transpire? You are still this physical self, and this energy needs to return back to life in some way. You go back *into* the world, but not *of* the world. You have your power to give and interchange, without becoming a slave to the world.

I have just recently begun to really study these pictures, and they say a lot to me. I want more of living it and being a part of it. In these past few days working with you we use words, we talk about our experience, and we also are a part of this experience of movement. I think the ox pictures also express your discipline in t'ai chi. You have your undisciplined body. You first *talk* about what you're doing and then you have a sense, "Ah! I feel my body going up, going down"—for the first time really physically and not just intellectually. Or you say, "Yes, when I push and grunt, I feel this energy." You begin to find harmony between what you say and what you experience. You can say, "Yes, now I feel exactly how it happens in my wrist and my elbow. Then there is the turning, the return, the turning around—Ah! my body comes around, faces me and says hello. My palm faces me and there is a relationship between us. There's a return, a continuation of this."

You gradually begin to have a sense of harmony and taming yourself, and it becomes more indescribable. You can follow the way and pretty soon you forget what you learned. You can really dance out of yourself; when you dance you feel like the cloud floating, soaking in the moonlight and letting it shine through you.

Tao te Ching

The *Tao te Ching* has been a very obscure book in this country until fairly recently because of the difficulty of understanding its meaning. The book consists of eighty-one short verses about the tao. It's very difficult to translate because of its paradoxes and puns, triple meanings and plays on words. The earliest translation appeared in Latin before 1800. There have been approximately thirty prominent English translations that I have seen. The most available ones are the versions by Legge and Waley and Blakeney. Lin Yutang also has a version, and there is a very poetic one by Witter Bynner. Gia-fu Feng and Jane English have recently created another. Most translators write a few pages of apology saying "I try my best, but you'll have to read the original text if you really want to understand it." The most you can do is to translate one way and then write a note and say, "It also can mean something else. I agree and do not agree. And also it can mean this, but perhaps not." Pretty soon you say, "Well, it's too obscure, too difficult for me to explain."

I began reading the *Tao te Ching* when I was a child. We used to sing and chant it and make it into rhymes. We learned it by sound and rhythm. We just learned how to pronounce the words and memorize them, but we didn't even know what most of them meant. This is how Chinese learn their classics, by repeated memorizing. Every morning you can hear school children chanting away, singing and just having fun with the sounds of the words. Maybe a few years later one day a passage from it suddenly means something to you. In high school I studied it again, and I thought I understood it. Then one day I looked at it and it didn't mean anything to me again.

Recently I've been practicing calligraphy again, and I make it a point to copy a few verses every day. I look at them and contemplate them, and let the characters and the meanings between the characters and between the strokes reveal themselves to me. Each time I copy the *Tao te Ching* I gain more insight into it, and that helps me to understand t'ai chi more clearly. All the philosophy and the imagery suggested in the book can be applied to our daily living.

The *Tao te Ching* is a very beautiful learning and meditation book. It is like a zen koan: either you dismiss it as nonsense, or you have to really dig in to understand it. It immediately takes you out of that intellectual confinement of getting stuck with ideas, with what you *think* you know. Much of it seems like nonsense if you translate it literally; but if you allow openness for all possibilities of each character, deeper meanings emerge. I hope you will receive my translations the way you would look at Chinese paintings in an art museum. Don't let the English explanations on the side of each picture confuse or limit your own intuitive understanding.

I find myself reluctant to interpret *Tao te Ching* to intellectuals who listen only with their heads. It is different with you. I have been moving with you, dancing with you, touching you. We have established a give-and-take communication. If we can spread all the words around, reshuffle their many meanings, and then let them settle, we may discover another way of perceiving this useful book.

I hope I will never think that I am a master of words and begin to believe that what I say is the truth. I will always have a problem talking, and making complete sentences in English. I fumble with my

I's and r's and plurals and singulars and past tense and future tense and genders. Steve has been saying it's fun transcribing my tapes because they *sound* very good. I understand what I'm saying when I hear it, but when I see the words written down, they look very funny. We've been joking about it, saying that this will be a pidgin-English translation.

The Chinese language has a very elusive quality. It never quite says it clearly. You want me to make absolute statements. All the *Tao te Ching* translations try to make clear sentences. But English grammar with its subject/object split can never express the tao. No translation will be adequate unless you really dig into the learning of Chinese—and most of you will not be able to do this in your lifetime. I have had the opportunity to know and explore tao in my practice of t'ai chi and calligraphy, so perhaps I can translate it in a way that will serve you in the same way as the work we have been doing this week. I just finished copying the *Tao te Ching* onto this scroll yesterday, so this will be a personal interpretation: what I see *now*, as I look at the characters on the scroll. I will only have time to translate the first fifteen chapters.

The very first chapter is one that you hear often when you begin to look into taoism. I will spend more time with it, to show you how many possibilities there are in translation. The first line is, "The tao that can be taoed is not the tao." We see three taos. The first tao is the noun tao, which is usually translated as "the way." The second tao is a verb which means to speak or to express. The third tao is also the noun, and with it is a character meaning "like always" or "natural." So we might translate it "The way that can be expressed is not the natural way." Or you could say, "The truth that can be expressed is not the eternal truth." Or, "The way that can be followed is not the ordinary way." You can also translate tao as path or road, so it could be "The path which can be shown is not the true path." So we already have many possibilities for the first six words. By the time you go through all the thirty-five or forty published variations, you feel the best way to say it is to stick with the original Chinese!

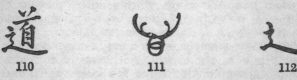

110   111   112

Another way to approach the *Tao te Ching* is to look deeply into the calligraphy as we did yesterday. The character for tao looks like this (110.). In the middle of the character there is a symbol of the center, the self (111.) which looks like a sketch of a primitive chief with deerhorn headgear. The lower part of the character (112.) looks like a path or a road. It also looks like water flowing or it could be a boat. So you might translate tao as "The path of the leader, that flows like water." Or you might say that it means "yourself, flowing with the way of nature." Or "If you walk on your own path, the natural spontaneous road, then you understand tao." The character is a circular, global concept of what tao is. You have to make your words connective and grasp it all together. So even within each character there are many possible translations.

The second line of the first chapter is very similar to the first: "The name that can be named is not the name." If you can name it and say "This is it," then you are wrong. One translation says "Existence is beyond the power of words to define." So right away we realize that the difficulty we have in pinning down a meaning to these characters is *exactly what the Tao te Ching is telling us*: the inability of words to fully describe what they attempt to describe, the inability of any teaching to show you the way.

The next part talks about being and non-being, existence and non-existence, the positive and negative, the yang and yin. "No-name is the beginning of heaven and earth. Name is the mother of all things." These two sentences are used as complements to each other. One says no-name is the origin of all things, and the other says name is. So again there is a paradox.

Next it says, "If you accept this paradox, the nature of existence, you can go on to contemplate its mystery." The character for mystery is composed of a woman and a child, which is used consistently throughout the book to mean the yielding yin and childlikeness. The character for contemplation looks like a crane standing in the water waiting for a fish, just resting there on long legs. It means awareness, or alertness, or observation.

"If you stay with non-being and follow it, then you will be able to sink into being in order to realize the completion of the mystery." This time we have a different character for mystery. This one is yang, to complement the yin character used earlier. When we try to describe this "mystery" with only the yin or the yang, we find ourselves speaking only part of the truth. If we realize that this mystery is a circle, then the essence is in the center, neither yin nor yang; it is in the union of the two polarities. "The two polarities come from the same source. You call it this; you call it that—but they are really the same thing. It's called the darker, or original mystery." This character for mystery suggests the color of dark silk, or the many layers of deep green inside dense woods. It's an elusive word to describe the tao. "Within the original mystery is a deeper mystery, and the gate opens."

When I try to translate *Tao te Ching* for you, I go through a helplessness of grabbing onto all the words I can find and then looking at your eyes and hoping that maybe when I say the "female," something clicks for you and you understand female. And when I say "child," somebody says "Child. Yes, that's the mystery for me." And "dark silk" adds another dimension. Finally I hope for a centering of all these bits and pieces into understanding.

2

The second chapter talks about comparison and judgment: "In this world, under heaven, when you point out and bring forth what is called beauty, *then* ugliness appears." The words beauty and ugliness in this sentence could also mean virtue and lack of virtue. When you know good, the bad appears. The minute you distinguish one thing as *such*, right away there is a comparison, and the opposite appears. In order to learn the tao, you must realize this. "Existence and non-existence, being and non-being, are two different sides of the same process; they are really mutually supporting each other. Difficulty and easiness construct each other's existence. The long and the short exist by comparison. Above and below are in relation, facing. Variations of sound have harmony. Forward and back follow each other."

Therefore, the man who understands tao, "the sage does by not doing; he teaches by practicing the wordless teaching." This character is usually translated as sage or wise man. Yesterday we had fun with this character's three roots: the listening ear, the speaking mouth, and the man centered between heaven and earth and connected to both. So rather than the wise man who *possesses* knowledge, it really means the person who *knows* tao and *flows* with tao. If you are a sage then you will create all things without feeling as if you have created them. "Give birth to events, but without pride or self-importance in the results. Act without interfering. When you succeed in achieving something or making something, do not linger or possess it. If you do not cling to your achievements, you will not lose them."

3

Certain chapters seem to be directed at those who have power over others. This is one of them. "If you do not favor talent, then the people will not fight for position. If you do not value things that are difficult to attain, then no one will steal or fight for them. If you do not show the desirable, then man's heart will not be confused trying to struggle for it. Therefore the sage rules by opening people's hearts and filling their bellies." This means to empty the mind of imagined desires and fulfill the natural needs. "The sage makes the people's ambition soft and gentle while strengthening their bones"—the structure that really holds us up. "If you let the people understand the true meaning of emptiness, *no*-knowledge, *no*-desires, then no one who wishes to know can interfere by trying to be or to do. By inaction, nothing is left undone."

4

"The tao seems to be very hollow and transparent and empty but when you *use* it, it's inexhaustible. It is very deep and mysterious. It's like the ancestor of all things. When you follow tao it will round off the sharp edges, untangle confusing threads, dim all glaring light. It molds and smoothes the dust." In Taoism, dust usually means the clutter in your mind: the inessential, bothersome little things that trouble us. "The tao unifies and brings together so that all the different thoughts become one."

"The tao is elusive in its beginnings. Sometimes you doubt its existence. We do not know whose son it is. It might be the offspring of gods who existed before all things."

5

"Heaven and earth are not benevolent; they treat all creatures as straw dogs." If we take this translation directly, it sounds negative. But in Chinese we know it really means "heaven and earth treat all things equally." We know that it is a paradoxical statement, stressing the unspoken as well as the spoken. The characters for heaven and earth used together mean the unknown, god. The character for benevolent is used in Confucianism to mean the relationship between two people. Straw dogs in China are used for sacrificial purposes. "The sage is not benevolent; he treats all men as straw dogs." The sage is also neither unkind nor kind. He practices inaction, and regards both men and straw dogs as part of the inclusive *all*. So there is no differentiation. Neither god nor sage makes judgments or distinctions. They allow all things to be spontaneous and realize their separate natures. "Between heaven and earth is like a bellows"—the hollow of a flute, or the inner space of a stone bell. Its emptiness allows all music to happen. "Its hollowness gathers more substance. The more the cycle of heaven and earth continues, the stronger it becomes. Too much speculation amounts to less—if you talk too much about it, you are really saying less. Stay in the middle of the truth."

6

"The spirit of the valley is immortal; we call it the mysterious cow." The cow represents the female essence. "The gate of the female mystery is the root of heaven and earth. It is like an endless fleecy cloud expanse, forever transforming. You may draw upon its effortless power without work or pain."

7

"Heaven is enduring. Earth is everlasting." Heaven and earth are infinite in time and space because "they do not give birth to themselves." They exist without the consciousness of self. "Therefore the sage, the man who flows with tao, puts his self in the back, and stays in front. By putting his self outside, therefore he exists inside." As in t'ai chi, "the best foot forward" really means that we yield back in order to advance. But the sage does not make a conscious effort to put his self last in order to stay front. "He realizes his self by being selfless."

8

"The highest virtue is like the nature of water. Water is beneficial to all things, but does not boast or fight to be so. Water runs to the lowest places, where no one wants to be. It is close to the tao." If you are like the water, then you will be at home in any environment. "Meditate into the depth of the heart. In relationship, give and take. In dialogue, be truthful and trusting." In modern Chinese printing of old classics, punctuation marks are inserted to help you read it easily. When I wrote this on the scroll, I intentionally left out all the punctuation so that I could read it in the old way. Hundreds of new possible interpretations can emerge, depending on how you group the words together. I will go on reading the rest of this chapter, character by character: "Center, goodness, control, serve, virtue, ability, movement, goodness, time, because, only, no, fight, therefore, no, blame." Let me now try to collect all these broken ideas. If you stay in the middle, then you know how to govern wisely. If you allow the person to act, then he develops his abilities. And if you know how to move, then you can take the timely opportunity. Because you do not fight or interfere with the nature of things, you do not have fear of resentment or blame.

9

"Better to remain unfilled, than carry around spilling. Sharpen weapons too much, and their sharpness cannot be long preserved. If you fill your house with gold and jade, you cannot keep it safe. If you boast of your knowledge and flaunt your possessions, you invite resentment and blame. When the work is done and it brings you honor, recede, not clinging to your achievement. This is the tao of heaven."

10

"Carry body and soul to embrace oneness; can you maintain their unity without separation? Concentrating on your ch'i, your vital breath, can you be soft and easy, like an infant child? Cleansing the unlimited vision, can you be without blemish? Love your people and govern your domain, can you be without effort and purpose? When the gate of the dark mystery, the yin, opens and closes, can you retain the yang, and fly toward it like a male bird? Illuminating your paths and clearing your four directions, can you reach your destination without pre-planned action? Give birth, nourish, but do not possess. Serve without self-con-gratulations. Nurture growth without control. This is the primal virtue of the tao."

11

"Thirty spokes make a wheel. But it's both the spokes and the space between them that is of use to the wagon. When you throw a pot it is both the clay and the space within that is useful. Build windows and doors. It is the space they create that gives use-fulness to them. Understand the advantage of having the exterior, but use the fertile void within."

12

"Five colors are blinding. Five sounds are deafen-ing. Five flavors dull your palate. Racing in the open field hunting for gain, one becomes crazy with de-sires. The more difficult the object is to obtain, the more man craves it and fears losing it. Therefore the sage satisfies the need in his belly, and closes his eyes to the superficial. Let go of *that*, outside yourself, retain *this*, inside yourself."

13

"Being favored and disgraced both bring fearful anticipation. Honor and misfortune are the normal conditions of the self. What is meant by fearful antici-pation? Being favored puts one in a vulnerable posi-tion. It's a surprise to receive favor; but fear of losing it leads to anguish. What is meant by normal conditions of honor and misfortune? I bring about my own misfortune because of my own self-interest. If I have no self, how could it have misfortune? Therefore, he who understands the cultivation of selflessness can be entrusted with the world."

14

"Look and you can't see it—it is the transparent. Listen and you can't hear it—it is the soundless. Grasp it and you lose it—it is the untraceable. These three are inseparable, therefore united as one. Above, its aura doesn't glare. Below, its humility is not obscure. Ongoing, everchanging, it can't be named. It once again circles back to nothingness. The formless form, the imageless image, it is flickering at you. When you meet it, you do not see its head; when you trail it, you do not see its tail. Follow the ancient tao to be *now*. Knowing the old beginning is the order of tao."

15

"The ancient man of tao was subtle, yielding, and childlike. His profound comprehension of the tao eludes us. Because it is beyond definition we must recognize it through metaphors:

Hesitant and alert, as if crossing a winter stream.

Watchful and aware, as if awaiting unexpected encounter from all sides.

Quiet and polite, as if a guest.

Dispersing and subdued, like ice melting away.

Simple and unpretentious, like the 'uncarved block.'

Open and receiving, like the broad valley facing up.

All embracing and unassuming, like muddy water.

How is it possible to absorb all impurities and remain untainted? By quiescence, just as cloudy water clears when it becomes still.

How can one maintain this quietude and peace? By allowing movement, like the ripples in the settling water.

He who preserves the secret of the tao lives without exceeding his own needs, content with what he has and what he is."

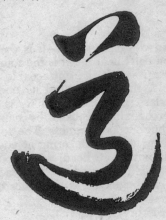

IX

I have noticed a great deal of extension and energy change during the week. Not just individually, but as a whole group. It's a really good feeling. I was comparing notes with another group leader last night during the dancing session. We were both sitting there sweating and smiling. He said, "This week has gone by so *fast*," and I said, "Yah. It's pretty much like one thing flowing into another." When you have to plan what to do next, or think, "What have we done?" "What needs improving?" then things begin to drag. Then you worry, and you wonder what happened. If we are very conscious that "This is the last session," then we have to make a special point to do something important. "I have to wrap it up." But I don't feel the need to close the circle. This space in the open end is useful.

There is a story of a man who goes to a taoist to seek enlightenment. One of the master's disciplines is pottery. After he has been with him for some time, he begins to feel that he understands. One day he picks up one of his master's pots to admire, and he drops it. He feels a tremendous sense of loss as the pot shatters. The taoist says, "Why? You don't need to be remorseful. It's still there." The enlightened master recognizes that it is not the pot that matters, but the experience of making it.

This week I have been spending most of my free time in my cabin, copying the *Tao te Ching*. Working on it refreshes me and dissolves whatever tension I have built up in my body from teaching. I have some anxiety because of my responsibility as a leader. It's obvious and I know it. One of my feelings about leading workshops is that as long as I am involved and doing it with you, I am also with me. I don't have to say, "All right, now it's *my* time," and dash back to the cabin and say, "Ahh, now I'm alone." T'ai chi teaches us not to have one face for giving and another for taking.

I made a big mistake yesterday when I talked about the *I Ching*. After we talked about the ox pictures and the *Tao te Ching*, the next thing in my plan was the *I Ching*. But I didn't prepare myself by simply writing the text and meditating on it the way I did with the ox pictures and the *Tao te Ching*. Instead I went into a real mind-trip of digging out information. Out of my own interest I got out all my Chinese books on the *I Ching* and made notes and lists. The more garbage I accumulated, the more intense and cluttered I got.

By the time we were gathered together again to talk I was stuffed with information that I wanted to give to you. But I was still just on the periphery of all this information which I hadn't yet resolved into real understanding. Yesterday's session became a real mental burden for me; I got exhausted.

And the interesting thing I learned was how observant you are becoming. I heard you saying, "Very interesting, Al. This is the first time I've noticed your hand shake as you do the brushwork." "Your voice seems to give up some of the easy flow." In contrast, this is what I heard from some of the outsiders who just sat in on that one session: "Wow, I certainly admire your *knowledge*. You *know* so much!" "I didn't understand a thing you were saying, but I certainly enjoyed it."

The moment that the mind starts to seek information for information's sake, the flow stops and you begin to function unnaturally. Anxiety shows, the muscles tense up, the shaking begins and you become

confused and cluttered. During the *I Ching* reading
I felt I was getting heavier and heavier. I was trying
to answer deep questions from my head instead of
from my tant'ien. I almost got us into a dead end.
When I realized we were getting bogged down, my
first urge was to get up and move. As soon as we did,
I sensed a feeling of ease and trust in the group
again. And then I had a feeling of "Ah, they are
people!" I realized how much I had been lecturing
and broadcasting, and how little I was in contact with
you.

When I discussed the imagery of the zen ox pictures, it came through me at that moment of interpretation—and the same was true of the *Tao te Ching*.
Nothing happened in the *I Ching* reading except feed-
ing you a lot of indigestible bits of unnecessary
information.

In a previous workshop I asked each person to go
into the woods each day for a quiet walk, and collect
yarrow stalks as he meditated on questions important
to him. On the last day we used the yarrow stalks to
demonstrate how the *I Ching* is used in China. I inter-
preted the hexagrams out of my experience at that
moment, reflecting our week of work/play together.
We had a really organic mind/body experience, instead of the usual head-heavy discussions.

We managed to lift the heaviness yesterday by
getting up to move. Then we began to let go and flow
more easily. Often when your mind is cluttered like
this you rationalize and say, "I don't feel like dancing." If your mind is not dancing, you don't feel like
dancing with your body. Whatever is in your mind is
jammed up, forcing, fighting. Sometimes the best way
is to allow the dancing body help sort out the sitting
mind. We know that we can affect the mind by working with the body, and we do it deliberately—this is
why we call t'ai chi a movement discipline. You cannot force inaction. But when you find yourself grinding your teeth and feeling all jammed up, you can begin a movement process that will eventually untangle
and unclutter your mind.

Whenever I feel weighed down, I use movement as my discipline. I begin to dance in my studio, and the interesting thing is that when I allow the t'ai chi way of moving to happen, I always end up dancing naturally, happily. The meaning of discipline to me is not something that is forced on you from outside—by a person, a book, or an idea—but by your own understanding and awareness of what serves you. When I dance and move, everything seems to fall in the right place for me.

Last night it took us a long time to get into the flow. In the previous sessions it happened very quickly because we had live music and many enthusiastic visitors joining in. There was a lot of energy going, and you could easily become a part of the rhythm. You didn't have any obligation to keep it up. You could step out to rest and drink your tea, or take a walk with the moon and the ocean, then come back whenever you felt like it and explore the rhythm that had developed. It was like a boiling pot. You could come in and have a bowl of soup whenever you wanted to. You didn't have to watch the boiling process. It was there, taking care of itself.

Last night we had a smaller group and only taped music, and we were more responsible for our own energy and helping it become part of the boiling process. It's much harder to dance and be a part of the dancing that way. The evening went on and on, and we tried different tapes and different things. Finally most people had left and I said this was the last tape. After the tape recorder was unplugged and put away, there was some singing going on. Paul was playing an autoharp. A young man started playing his bamboo flute. I was going to get my coat, but it wasn't there, so I started dancing. And Nancy started dancing. And Roger started dancing. Sidney was lying there, taking off her belt, flinging it to the side and letting her whole body go, and she started singing lying down. Suddenly we formed a circle, moving like fire, and I said, "*This* is the real beginning."

It took us the whole evening. In spite of ourselves

pushing, rushing, and losing that true feeling, finally we reached it again. If we stay with that process long enough, we become it. So much is happening this week—the way you move, the way you feel, the way you look—that pleases and surprises you. And I must say as I look at you from day to day there is a new twinkle in your eye. The way you walk and the way you take the ground is more solid. When I come to you and touch your hand, it slides out beautifully. I put my arm around your back and feel you flowing more and more. I would like to work a little bit more just to bring everything into the flow, so we can circle back and then let the structure disappear.

I want to first work with the stance. There's a tendency when you are in the beginning stage of t'ai chi to be so concentrated on the upper body movement that you get very tight in your stance. Put your hands right over your thigh muscles, above your knees. If you twist around you can feel how the muscles move and flow.

If you have kinks or tightness somewhere in your body, instead of trying to pull that area open and stop everything else, just try to let it flow into the rest of your body. The t'ai chi way of loosening up is to let movement make easy connections. Before I understood this, I always used to have muscle pain and tightness in my thighs the day after a dance performance. Now when I dance well, my body feels twice as good the next morning.

Now pivot and move around a little bit. Explore the footwork. You see how I walk in the morning when I do my sword practice. You may think I am copying Toshiro Mifune, the Japanese actor who often plays the samurai. Actually I am taking my time feeling the stone slabs or the boards under my feet. If one of the boards is loose or broken, I should be able to shift to a new base instantaneously. Look underneath you now as you move, and imagine that down deep is a dungeon or a bottomless pit. This seemingly safe floor may suddenly crumble. Be tentative, sensing, ready to shift your base if the floor gives way. Imagine that you are stepping on thin ice about to break, or rocks are moving underneath you as you cross a creek. If something changes beneath your feet, can you re-adjust quickly and easily? Learn to accept the fact of insecurity as a norm. You can relax and find security on top of insecurity. Alan Watts has a book called *The Wisdom of Insecurity,* and he wanted to call one of his workshops here "Shangri-la at the edge of the San Andreas fault." Esalen didn't want to emphasize the earthquake possibility so they changed the title to "Shangri-la at the edge of the sea," and it became meaningless.

Insecurity and uncertainty are everywhere. If you don't let it become part of your flow, you will always be resisting and fighting. If the ground here suddenly shakes and trembles, can you give with it and still maintain your center? The joy in surfing and skiing and so many other sports is in being able to do this. If you stiffen up and fight the wave, then you will never learn; you have to give in to the waves in order to ride them. If you can become fluid and open even when you are standing still, then this fluidness and openness makes you able to respond to changes. You will be able to play with the changes and enjoy them.

Here's another image to get that feeling of re-silience into your base. Imagine that you are a bird hopping from one twig to another. Move from one spot to another as if you are landing on a very re-silient branch that bends and bounces in response to your weight. Don't jump with both feet; hop onto it with one foot, and then bring your other foot lightly underneath you. You should have a sense of compact-ness, of sinking your weight gently onto that bounc-ing twig. If this branch is in the wind, then the branch is moving you. You have to give in and obey like the branch that responds to the wind.

At the same time you are not rooted to that twig; you are ready to hop to another if this twig isn't strong enough to support you. With each step, test the re-silience and unevenness and the weight of your stance. Instead of trusting that particular spot to support you,

you can trust your own flowing base. Then you never have that insecure, grabby feeling.

Now as I come around and push you, see if you can maintain your center by adjusting your base. Don't plan what to do, just maintain an openness and fluidity, so that you can yield to the force instead of fighting it. Receive the energy right down into your center and down into your moving base.

You can do so much if you keep your base and your center. If you jump on me and wrap close around my hips like a snake, I can carry you easily regardless of your weight, because I am carrying you close to my center. Pair up with someone about your size and try this. Move around and pivot, and feel how much weight you can carry at your center. After you have done this, move around individually and feel your own weight in the same way. Embrace yourself the way you just embraced the other person.

At the same time that you are aware of yourself and your base, be aware of the space around you, as if you are a samurai with attackers coming from all sides. Your base is like a smooth, calm, spinning motion. In an instant you can face all directions and ward off your attackers—"Tsa! Hunh! Anh!" The sound is not a separate thing, it's part of the extension of your movement. Sometimes it may not be audible, but the sound is there if the throat is free, if the breathing is free. It's like singing when you dance. It makes good sense to sing as you dance. In most folk-dancing the song and the movement really fit together. When you vocalize with a movement like this, you express what you feel deep down in your body.

Another good reason for making sounds is that you get so involved with them that you have no time to mess up your functioning. There is no time for thinking out your opponent's moves and planning what you will do next; you maintain your energy and remain open and flexible until the exact moment of encounter. It is also a powerful display to show your readiness and courage. But mainly we use it as a very creative and playful expression of primitive energy that comes from way down here in your belly, the tant'ien. It's a reminder of where your center is.

During my sword practice this morning a cat came running towards me. She pulled back just beyond the tip of my sword and cautiously walked all around me. Then she sat very alert and motionless waiting for my next move. After I finished, I walked over to the edge of the deck where lots of other cats were playing and stretching, waiting, pausing, pouncing, suspended—centered and sensing each other's energy. They were doing the exact thing I had been practicing. This alertness is being completely here and centered, ready to move and react to the instant. The drop of a pin will affect you—not to make you jump and sweat nervously, but simply alert you.

T'ai chi definitely connects you with whatever is happening around you. In Antonioni's documentary film on China *Chung Kwo* (the middle kingdom) one sequence showed a busy city intersection during the morning rush hour. There was an old man swiftly riding his bicycle to work—going through his t'ai chi motifs with his arms and torso. He was doing his morning meditation, yet obviously fully aware of the hectic traffic surrounding him.

Now let's review some of the things we've been working with. Settle down, and just let the body go. Feel a plumb line that goes straight through the middle of you, very close to the spine. If you are standing with your legs too close together, or too wide apart, the plumb line will be weakened. Your legs should be directly underneath your hips. The correct stance for t'ai chi gives you a nice open parallel feeling, so you don't feel uneven. The shoulders are dropping downwards because of the gravity of your arms going down, but this dropping does not make the back bend. The back is going upward, with the awareness of each disc on top of the next. Feel the space between the discs growing in an upward lift.

The weight in the shoulders flows downward so that it gives you a sense of floating. It's a settling weight, not a supported weight; that makes the difference. Think of a stone dropping through water. The stone sinks and the water doesn't try to support the stone. Allow your shoulders to sink into your base like a stone dropping through water.

If you are still holding the elbows up, let them go in the same way. Let the elbows be pulled down by your forearms and fingertips. Allow your chest to be hollowed instead of sticking out. Don't make a special point of being concave but let go of all that "chin up, chest out" forward look of your posture that is usually drummed into you. Work on the whole feeling of sinking, pulling down, hollowing, emptying. Let it fall through the thigh into the kneecap and let go of the kneecap into the calf, into your ankle, all the way down into your root, your base. Keep rooting down without being nailed and stuck.

At the same time that you let the body sink, you still keep an upward feeling in the spine. There is a spot here at the crown of your head that can help you to keep the upward motion going. Feel it extend toward the ceiling, and beyond the ceiling into the space above. So you have this sense of upwardness, and you also have the sense of downwardness. You have the sense of expansion with the breath in your torso, and a sense of pulling up between your legs into the center line of your body. Let the body give in to the legs, and let the knees go, in order to allow the pivoting movement as you turn. All that comes together, and then you float on top of it.

Remember that the face is part of your body. Unlock your jaw, and let your lips come slightly apart. Release your thinking by releasing the tongue in your mouth. Let the tongue float, with the top of your tongue gently touching the palate, like an open valve. The jaw is very important because any tightness here stiffens your neck and restricts your head movement. The looseness of the facial parts is very important.

When you practice t'ai chi, you may wish to begin with your eyes closed, to get the feeling of your body. But when you start to move, look ahead without any tension. If you *try* to hold your eyes open, then you will have the urge to blink. Just let your vision go out and spread around and slope down. Think of the peripheral vision going out both sides and curving around. Don't wear horse blinders so you don't see anything to the side of you.

You must also use your ears. Let all sounds come into you without resisting or letting any of them bother you. Don't categorize them. Don't say, "That's the ocean—that's bird—that's him talking—that's kitchen—that's footsteps." If you keep identifying things specifically, then you become partial. Just allow yourself to sense everything, and to go through the whole emptying, relating process.

This can be a frustrating stage when you're learning to practice t'ai chi. When we dance, when we just improvise, we can rely on the rhythm of the music to help us to let go. Now, you have to learn to rely on your own sensing and energy. Like any really exciting thing that happens spontaneously, it has to begin simply. When you practice t'ai chi in the morning, I want you to be patient with this.

Pay attention to the circular movement of your breathing. Allow the breathing pattern to really circulate inside of you, inside of your torso. Let it flow into your arms, up to your neck, to the top of your head, and down the backbone into your legs. Then energy can begin to expand to all directions at once. Feel all the energy from outside coming towards you, and your energy reaching out as your arms begin to lift. The rising of your arms is balanced by a sinking into your base, as the energy of the circle expands. Think of an expansion instead of a cut-and-dried hand-lift and knee-bend. Try this first movement several times. Think of that expansion into all directions from the center of your body and then the coming together, the collecting back to straight upright center support. Let that feeling of energy open you out into a curving yin/yang intertwining up/down flow as you expand in your arms and settle into your base. Then the outward energy curves and turns inward as your arms sink and your pelvis rises and you return to center.

This energy must be a part of you; you must never move as an objective outsider observing. You must always be inside of it, with it. This is the only way you can do t'ai chi.

When you prepare for the beginning of your t'ai chi, you first allow your stance to become uneven until it begins to settle into evenness. Then you begin to sense the space all around you, including the space that's beyond the floor. This way you will feel that you are suspended in the middle of a sphere of energy. As you move, you play with this energy that comes from all sides. You play with the horizontal curve, the vertical curve, the slanting curve, the curve beneath you and above you—all over, all around.

In China you would have to practice this beginning movement for many months before the master would allow you to do anything else. There is a good reason for this. In the beginning you are fragmented. You think about your wrist, or maybe your elbow; you think of the knee and then you think of the spine. You do serial things, because your experience is still in bits and pieces. When you really get a sense of doing this movement, it all happens simultaneously. You sense all events, all the directions, all the energies going, without having to consciously direct your attention to your wrist or elbow or shoulder. It all happens together: a sense of time, personal connection— one on-going, flowing, immediate sequential flash.

So when you practice t'ai chi in the morning, just do this first movement for a while. It's *plenty* to work on. You only get bored if you focus on the outside, the peripheral, instead of the inside, the essential. If I put it very simply t'ai chi is this one movement— that's all.

Now, let t'ai chi happen and let the essence take over. Embrace Tiger, Return to Mountain: The first and the last and all major variations of this one movement will develop slowly like waves moving in and rolling out. Recall the different ways you have been practicing breathing with this circular motif. Reach outward to embrace all the energy around you. Your arms gather in, cross, and lift up to about chest level, and then you relax your elbows and let your hands revolve. Then gently push all this energy down into your tant'ien—Return to Mountain. Let your arms return to rest at your sides as all this energy settles and simmers down. Keep flowing through. Remember the sensation of the stone falling into water, with your elbows drooping and pulling down. Your chest feels hollow, the tongue is loose, touching the palate gently; the breathing passages are open. Just keep feeling the energy moving within your stillness.

The change of energy curves, the level curves. There is no stopping and beginning; it's on-going. You are very steady. You feel very constant and very still as you move, and you feel the motion within your stillness. Movement and stillness become one. One is not a static point. One is a moving one, one is a changing one, one is everything. One is all the movement you can possibly do with the human body. One is also that stillness suspended, flowing, settling, in motion. You do not stand still now in contrast to your moving around. All the energy that you can possibly use in the whole spectrum of your expression is settling, contained within this form of t'ai chi. It is not a confinement or elimination of the rest of your energy levels and your energy varieties, but they must be connected to become this one feeling.

Wherever you are, whatever you do, you can always come back to this marvelous sense of stillness, the feeling of yourself, very, very much *here*. This is your reference point; this is your stability. This is your life force that gives you balance. This is your home you carry around with you wherever you are. This is your powerhouse, your reservoir, your endless inexhaustible resource, that center you that is teaching and sharing and working with all of us these past few days. And the movement goes on and on and on.

Afterword

Soon after this book began, Barry and Steve also found Shura. Barry asked me what Shura would be in Chinese: My brush answered, "Wave follows wave follows wave." Waves continue to form and follow one another, as our mutual learning and sharing move on.

Besides Pauline Oliveros, I want to mention two other composer friends of mine who are particularly successful in their creative synthesis of the music of East and West: Mantle Hood's *Owari* and *Emergence* and Chou Wen-chung's *Cursive* and *Riding the Wind*.

In my current teaching of Oriental Theatre, the actors utilize the ch'i energy to inner-direct their emotional rhythms and movement patterns. The tao is revealed vividly in simple exercises such as these: "I don't want you. (tant'ien) . . . I DON'T WANT YOU! (fire—water) . . . Are you going? (wood circle) . . . Let's talk first. (Return to mountain)." The ch'i takes care of our action and spontaneity. Learning dissolves and techniques become invisible.

Lark grows from an infant to a toddler during the course of this book. To observe her is t'ai chi itself. She teaches me daily that life is simple. Not long ago she demonstrated to me how easy it was to work the old toilet handle by jiggling it gently. Last summer, visiting the Stevenses at Shura, waking up at dawn in Barry's cave, I saw a small figure sitting cross-legged on the mat, transfixed, gazing into the eastern horizon —suddenly, Buddha woke up in me.

Suzanne reflects my day-to-day inconsistancies: "You must not be as centered as you think you are." "Your teaching certainly hasn't affected you." The ego-me becomes furious; the real me accepts. What one knows and can say to others often has little to do with what one really is. As I proof-read the final draft of the manuscript, I begin learning t'ai chi all over again. I get excited about the ideas and become involved with the practice, forgetting that *I* actually said it, did it and knew it, once. Wisdom is. It is not mine or yours to keep. Recognizing it intellectually is only the beginning of learning. The great learning happens with the experience that fulfills and renews as life moves on.

As I meditate on the yin-yang symbol, the perfect s-shape division becomes increasingly lopsided and uneven—it shifts and changes. If we insist upon the absolute perfection of the unaltered balance as designed on paper, very soon it will look like the cut-and-dried half/half, black/white split. Even an open concept is reduced to cliché by overwork and loses its real meaning. I propose a return to the ancient tao, the original t'ai chi before names, labels and divisions. Tao cannot be monopolized or patented. Call it WU CHI, the no-t'ai chi school of t'ai chi, similar to the no-sword swordsmanship and no-knowledge wisdom.

During one of our most frustrating editing sessions with the book, Suzanne and I made a vow to take the first printed copy in our hands, and toss it into the fire page by page to warm our bellies on a cold night, and simply let the ch'i glow.

AL CHUNG-LIANG HUANG

Maple, Ontario, Canada
September, 1973

ABOUT THE AUTHOR

AL CHUNG-LIANG HUANG grew up in the villages of China where he received his training in the classics and a variety of Oriental fine and martial arts. He later came to America to become an architect and a concert performer. He has taught theater/dance and body-mind synthesis of the Asian creative arts throughout North America and the Far East. He is currently the director of Lan T'ing Institute, affiliated with the Alan Watts Society for Comparative Philosophy in Sausalito, California. His other books are *Tao: The Watercourse Way* (as collaborator), *Dancing Brushes* (with photographs by Si Chi Ko) and *The Original Faces Before You Were Born* (with Richard Grossman). He is also the subject of a beautiful T'ai Chi film by Kai de Fontenay Productions.

The MS READ-a-thon needs young readers!

Boys and girls between 6 and 14 can join the MS READ-a-thon and help find a cure for Multiple Sclerosis by reading books. And they get two rewards—the enjoyment of reading, and the great feeling that comes from helping others.

Parents and educators. For complete information call your local MS chapter, or call toll-free (800) 243-6000. Or mail the coupon below.

Kids can help, too!

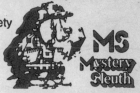